THE
'D' WORD

RETHINKING DEMENTIA

To all my past clients who have taught me
so much about caring.

Mary

This book is dedicated to all the people that I have met
over the years living well with dementia and proving
that the 'D' word doesn't have to be the final word.

To Yvonne and Craig Moss for all their care to Max.

Noel

THE
'D' WORD
RETHINKING DEMENTIA

MARY JORDAN
AND
DR NOEL COLLINS

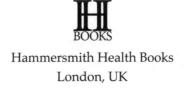

Hammersmith Health Books
London, UK

First published in 2017 by Hammersmith Health Books – an imprint of Hammersmith Books Limited
4/4A Bloomsbury Square, London WC1A 2RP, UK
www.hammersmithbooks.co.uk

British Library Cataloguing in Publication Data: A CIP record of this book is available from the British Library.

Print ISBN 978-1-78161-114-2
Ebook ISBN 978-1-78161-115-9

Commissioning editor: Georgina Bentliff
Edited by Carolyn White
Cover design and typesetting by: Sylvia Kwan
Cover image: Chris Jordan, reproduced *in memoriam*
Index: Dr Laurence Errington
Production: Helen Whitehorn, Pathmedia
Printed and bound by: TJ International Ltd

Contents

Acknowledgements

Many people have been involved in the writing of The 'D' Word. Those who played the biggest part were, once again, the people I have met who are living with dementia (either with a diagnosis or as carers and supporters) who gave the practical stimulus to my input. This book is written for them. I would like to thank Professor Peter Tyrer, FMedSci, for his discussions with me about the idea of using nidotherapy for people with dementia. My thanks also go to Dr Gillian Nienaber, BA Hons, BSc Hons, CinPsychD, who has given me constant help and facilitated expansion of my knowledge and experience of dementia.

My Editor, Georgina Bentliff, has, as always, given excellent technical support as well as wise encouragement and been endlessly patient with me. My sons and daughter-in-law have helped in the way that only close family can.

Mary, 2017

I would like to thank Mary and Georgina for all their expert advice and encouragement, and Carolyn for her expert editing. Also many thanks must go to Keith and Rosemary for their eagle-eyed critique of draft chapters. Lastly, I thank my husband Alberto, for his patience in living with The 'D' Word over the last year and his unstinting love and support.

Noel, 2017

Foreword

Since being diagnosed in 2010 with young-onset Alzheimer's disease, I have read very many books on the subject, using the adage that for me information is power, in this case over 'Dr Alzheimer' who resides inside my brain and from time to time causes some considerable mischief. Books I read in the early days were either focused on academics or on carers, and if a lay person wrote a foreword or preface it was usually a carer – most often one who had recently sadly lost their loved one after a traumatic end of life. Increasingly, with earlier and more accurate diagnosis, and with better post-diagnostic support and interventions, the voice of people like me is now being heard. Moving this forward, what we need are more and better examples of co-production and professionals writing with real insight and sensitivity, and that is what we have, I am delighted to say, within this book.

The 'D' Word presents two distinct yet entwined perspectives on what dementia entails for those living with the condition from two professionals who seek to deliver person-centred care. Noel clearly explains the science with insight and personal experience in order to help readers navigate their way without losing sight of the fact it is people who are at the centre of the issue, not statistics, numbers, service users, carers or patients. Alongside this, Mary draws from, and comments upon, a wealth of experience largely in the 'third sector' (voluntary/unpaid) which is increasingly being called upon to support people affected by dementia after diagnosis through a range of interventions.

I have known Noel for a little more than four years. We first met at a conference for the British Psychological Society and the Alzheimer's Society, and I was taken by his approach to de-mystifying the medical science around dementia and to challenging some widely held views by some of his colleagues in psychiatry. Following this we served together for two years on the Executive Committee of the Faculty for the Psychiatry of Old Age, where he helped a mere mortal like me to make some hopefully useful contributions. When he shared the thoughts about writing a book and for me to be involved he resisted the trap that many fall into by way of sending me a few samples to read and then write about. Noel actually came to my house and met with me to discuss the concept and contents of the book when it was still being written. He asked for my thoughts and advice and over a glass of Aussie red some lively conversation was conducted between us. Then, when the book was in draft, it was left to me how much I wanted to receive and how it could be best sent to me – paper rather than electronic so I could read it and annotate the text. Noel did all of this. I share this with you, the reader, because what I have described is very rare, and should not be; I am therefore delighted to share some thoughts on what will be a fundamental text in the library of books available on dementia.

At first, the choice of the title, *The 'D' Word*, puzzled, concerned and challenged me as I would not want people to refrain from using the word dementia in the way that people have shifted from using 'the C word' to talking openly about cancer. But then I know too well there are many people who are either service providers or service users who still fear the stigma which is so often attached to dementia and who use words like 'memory problem' to avoid its use. I do hope that this book will go some way to helping address this.

Seldom does a week pass that dementia fails to appear in

the national media, usually with a headline around a so-called wonder drug or the failures of our care system. Consequently, it is not surprising that dementia is regarded as the most feared health condition in the over-40 demographic. This book examines in depth factors around this and goes on to state that this need not be the case if understanding, compassion and appropriate care and support are available to people. I know from lived experience that living well with dementia is a double-edged sword, something to strive for and encourage while also being aware that it is not always possible and that then the emotional and psychological consequences of feeling that one is failing are often substantial. One lives with dementia and those closest to us live with us and what the condition brings with it. Everyone is different and this in a way makes the medical model, where symptoms and treatments can be prescribed or carried out to restore one's health, less successful in connection to dementia. In this book the authors have critically examined the medical and care aspects of dementia alongside a comprehensive analysis of what has justifiably been called the biggest challenge to health and social care in this country, and beyond.

To close, I absolutely commend *The 'D' Word* to you whether you are a professional working with those of us who are affected by dementia, a person with the condition or someone who cares for us, or someone who at the moment is looking in from the outside. There is something within this book to support, inform, challenge and then inspire you all.

Keith Oliver
Kent & Medway NHS Trust Service User Dementia Envoy
Alzheimer's Society Ambassador

Preface

In a time of five-minute news cycles, the internet, blogs and social media, we encounter stories of life on a daily basis. In lifestyle pages, there are often articles regarding infidelity, the benefits of vitamin D, prison conditions, sexuality, breast-feeding, pensions and the benefits of yoga in motherhood. Mundane facets of life are constantly examined and discussed. Very occasionally, dementia makes headlines. Invariably these centre on the 'impending epidemic', the latest promise of a cure or a shocking story of abuse in a nursing home. There is rarely any discussion of memory, memory loss and how cognitive impairment and dementia will be part of our future – either directly or through someone we know. It seems discussion of dementia, like the other D-word – death – is studiously avoided.

Rather than talking about dementia throughout life, we hope it will affect someone else and only think of it when it becomes a reality. We need to change this and adopt a new approach, both on an individual level and as a society. We can learn from approaches to other topics to enlighten discussion of dementia. The disability movement in particular has been vital in shifting discussions of disability away from individual impairment to a more accessible social environment for all. But for any similar dementia movement to emerge, people must be willing and able to talk about dementia more openly, particularly people living with cognitive impairments themselves.

HOW THIS BOOK AROSE

This book arose out of five years of conversations between ourselves, Mary and Noel, in our joint work in a memory clinic in Surrey. For several years the local Community Mental Health Team had worked closely with dementia support workers from the Alzheimer's Society to offer people newly diagnosed with dementia support following diagnosis. Due to a change in location of the memory clinic to a small room in the outpatients' department of a regional hospital, the only way that we could work together was to physically sit together in the same room and see patients together. It turned out to be a serendipitous arrangement, although initially both of us were unsure that it would work. We thought that patients would prefer a private consultation with the psychiatrist, and so naturally every new patient was offered the opportunity to object to having the dementia support worker present. We discovered, though, that people were generally pleased that the medical services were enlightened enough to involve the third sector support services. People also only had to share their story once.

Most people who attended the clinic were referred by their local doctor, and had a history of memory problems. Our job was to diagnose dementia and support people after the diagnosis. This typically involved talking to the 'patient' and their family about their symptoms and relevant history, performing a memory test, and reviewing and ordering investigations (such as brain scans and blood tests). An assessment was then made about whether a patient had dementia or not, and if they did, which type and whether treatment with a cognitive enhancer (medication) could be offered. Practical advice would also be given about issues such as housing, driving, lasting power of attorney and advance care directives, and people were given information about further support and services.

As we felt our way forward in this joint way of working

several things became clear. The first feedback we had – from the people we were trying to help – was upbeat and positive. People told us that they were delighted at being offered a 'joined up service'. There were other important outcomes. We both learned a great deal from each other. Over time we came to realise that the close co-operation between our two services filled a 'missing link' in what was on offer to those now living with dementia.

We saw that a traditional medical approach could only offer people with dementia (PwD) certain answers to certain questions, and support services could only offer a part solution to managing dementia. Increasingly, we noted that when we looked beyond the biology to the social context of the PwD, a more positive and helpful approach emerged. We found that we naturally became more curious about the lives of the people we saw, and discovered that many of the answers surrounding the question of how to live well with dementia were being provided by the PwD themselves. We received as much wisdom from PwD and their carers as we attempted to deliver. We witnessed, at first hand, people managing the challenge of dementia with creativity, humour, determination and dignity. And we were impressed at how many people living with dementia, and their families and friends, intuitively adapted their worlds to make them more dementia-friendly. Conversely, we noted how many people struggled from day one to make sense of their or their loved one's condition, and felt let down at every turn by a system perceived to be uncaring and inflexible.

This book attempts to crystallise some of this wisdom and to pose a number of questions about how society can normalise, accommodate and even embrace the experience of dementia, as a natural consequence of us living longer lives, rather than it being feared as an epidemic of a soul-destroying disease.

We decided early on to keep each to our own perspective and write about the different aspects of dementia in the same way that we worked together in the memory clinic. So, in this book, each chapter addresses a different aspect, with each area considered from a clinician's point of view and from a more pragmatic 'what to do' viewpoint. We attempt to characterise the barriers and societal restraints that prevent everyone from finding some peace in their dementia experience. People fear a life or a death without meaning. Dementia does not directly cause this. It is, we have found, the way that society views and processes PwD that causes real disability and distress. This book is a conscious attempt to highlight some of these processes and provide some pragmatic advice to anyone touched by dementia so that they can feel more empowered in their situation, despite the absence of a cure. Our chapters are arranged around the broad themes that we found underpinned difficulties frequently experienced by people living with dementia. In each, we also muse on possible responses and solutions.

The aim of the book is not to politicise the reader, but, any discussion of dementia must touch on politics. People in the latter stages of their lives, with or without dementia, are particularly vulnerable to the effects of social policy. One of the reasons for this is that socioeconomic conditions in later life reflect the cumulative effect of life choices and circumstances over the entire lifespan. Many older people live their lives in relative poverty at a time where they may have to rely on health and social care systems for the first time in their lives. Mary and I noted, time and time again in our clinic, that people were often completely unaware of the complexities of the health and social care systems until they were suddenly forced to navigate both in a time of crisis. There was often a rude awakening as PwD and their families were exposed to the realities of means-tested adult social care. There was also sudden exposure to the stark differences in funding and assessment between health and social care and the difficulties in trying to broker care packages or nursing home placements in the private sector. People are often surprised that overworked and underfunded local authorities can only offer limited advice and financial support in a time of crisis. And in many cases, families had to find and fund their own solutions to complex problems.

Managing expectations became a key part of our job in our memory clinic. We frequently acknowledged that whilst the UK was good at producing aspirational mission statements regarding good and accessible care in dementia, such as the national carer and dementia strategies and the Wanless review of funding of adult care,[1] the reality of trying to organise and fund care for a loved one with dementia remained very difficult for many. In particular, brokering care for an adult with dementia in a crisis remains a huge challenge to families.

We remain convinced that the biggest real source of stress to PwD and their families after diagnosis is not the absence of a 'magic bullet' or cure, but the worry about the provision of future care. In particular, how good care can be obtained, maintained and paid for. For the very wealthy, this is less of a concern, but for everyone else, this is a significant source of stress. We write this just after the release of another UK chancellor's statement, and a clear absence of any policy to address an impending care crisis. There is now a perfect storm emerging that will threaten adult care provision in the UK. There is a lack of money, a lack of staff and a lack of policy. This, combined with a societal obsession with risk mitigation and paternalism, is a toxic threat to those in receipt of adult care. We fear that PwD, one of the most vulnerable groups in society, will be most affected.

SOCIOLOGY AND THE SOCIOLOGY OF DEMENTIA

It is perhaps important at this point to state one of the author's [Noel's] ideological leanings. When any medical student starts a psychiatric course, they are exposed to the 'bio-psycho-social' formulation. This suggests that any presentation, be it depression or psychosis or a memory problem, can potentially be addressed by considering a range of biological, social and psychological factors, the emphasis being that it is important to consider all three domains in any given psychiatric problem. Over the course of my professional life, I have tried to improve my skills in all three areas. I have obtained postgraduate qualifications in the biological (geriatric medicine) and the psychological (cognitive behavioural psychotherapy) and developed an interest in social contact and housing as the foundation for any good health. Several diplomas later, I still felt that there was something missing. In 2015, I enrolled in a Masters programme at King's College London to study gerontology. This is the study of ageing, not just from a biological perspective but also from the social, cultural, legal, political and economic point of view, looking at how these factors interact to affect the experience of ageing and later life.

The discipline of gerontology has much to offer in understanding the experience of dementia. Although the diseases of dementia are linked to specific pathological changes in the brain, the lives of PwD are as much affected by the society and social structures around them, such as health and social care, economic policy, socioeconomic and legal status and the broader culture. If we critically examine these factors, we can see what needs to change to help PwD live more fulfilling lives, in terms of social policy but also around societal values regarding memory, autonomy and personhood. This is important as I think it is unlikely that a 'cure' will ever be found (for reasons that will be explained in the book). However, if we can reconnect with our basic humanity, adopt a more holistic view of our worth, and challenge rigid assumptions regarding the relationship between the self and memory, then the search for a 'cure' for dementia is less desperate than it would initially seem.

I am not for a second disparaging the tireless efforts of scientists looking for biological tools in fighting dementia, I am suggesting that a more critical examination of the social experience of dementia should be explored in parallel with the search for a medical breakthrough. I am arguing, in a sense, for a duality in dementia care, whereby we can accommodate not only biological concepts of disease and treatment, but also an appreciation of the societal and other broader contexts and meanings important in the dementia experience.

This is in keeping with a bio-psycho-social approach where all dimensions of a disease are utilised to help the affected individual. Mary and I found this happy medium in our work together, in that we offered a sociological frame of reference alongside a more traditional biomedical approach. We believe this to be a more empowering response. This is because, although dementia is biological entity, it is also a social experience.[2] People with dementia and their carers live in a social reality, rather than a biological one. And whilst the biology of dementia may not be changeable, the way we relate as individuals to PwD, is. Whilst funding and support for research into biomedical interventions and potential cures for dementia are important, policy makers should not put all their eggs in one basket. The search for a cure should not displace a critical examination of how we care for PwD. And in particular, how we can enable a PwD to find meaning in their experiences and maintain their personhood and quality of life, irrespective of the condition.

THE VISION

The vision of this book is to enable PwD and their carers realise they have more control over their situation than they may think. We also hope to emphasise that it is not PwD who need to change, but rather society that needs to adjust as the number of those with dementia and cognitive impairment grows steadily in number. For society to become truly dementia-friendly, it needs to consider all angles of the dementia question. What are the benefits and limits of pursuing a medical model? Is memory the most important issue in dementia? How does one maintain a sense of self and personhood successfully? How can the diagnosis of dementia be used alongside the person? Is it more helpful to consider dementia a cognitive disability rather than a disease? What is the true nature of care in dementia? How can one live an authentic emotional life in dementia? What is 'mindful' dementia? Are their benefits of dementia? What are the politics of dementia, particularly within the nursing home? How can one successfully navigate the seas of health and social care? How can one die well with dementia? What is the future of dementia and 'cognitive disability'? This book attempts to provide some answers and encourage more debate around the dementia question.

This book is not intended to be a textbook of dementia, nor does it claim any definitive approach to the condition. Its main aim is to wrestle the narrative away from traditional biomedical viewpoints of deficit, decay and neurodegeneration and encourage more conversation and shared learning about the social experience of dementia. We need to re-appropriate the 'D' word. We hope that by rethinking dementia from sociological and other perspectives, PwD can be supported as individuals living their lives with cognitive disability rather than just being seen as helpless victims of a senile epidemic. We also hope that caring in dementia can achieve more status and become more valued as one of the best examples of humanity, rather than being viewed as a terrible burden in an individualistic society where autonomy is highly prized. We hope that PwD will become more visible and retain their full citizenship in a more dementia-friendly society. And we hope that this endeavour captures the imagination of society as a whole. We do not see ourselves as the custodians of knowledge here. However, we hope that the sharing of our experience and thoughts garnered whilst working together with hundreds of PwD may help others live well with the condition.

Mary Jordan and Dr Noel Collins
2017

REFERENCES

1. Wanless D, Forder J, Fernández J-L, Poole T, Beesley L, Henwood M, et al. *Wanless Social Care Review: Securing Good Care for Older People: Taking a Long-term View*. London: Kings Fund; 2006.

2. Beard RL, Knauss J, Moyer D. Managing disability and enjoying life: How we reframe dementia through personal narratives. *Journal of Aging Studies*, 2009;23(4): 227-35.

About the Authors

Mary Jordan is an independent trainer in dementia and related subjects having worked for many years for one of the major UK dementia charities; before that she had first-hand experience of dementia, both through caring for friends and relatives, and professionally. She also has many years of experience working for the National Health Service. In addition to articles and papers published in medical, nursing and social care journals and general magazines, Mary is best known for her books *The Essential Carer's Guide*, *The Essential Carer's Guide to Dementia*, the award-winning *End of Life*, *The Essential Guide to Caring* and *The Essential Guide to Avoiding Dementia*.

Dr Noel Collins is an older adult psychiatrist serving GP practices based in Haringey, London. Much of his community work relates to diagnosing memory problems and delivering appropriate treatment for patients with dementia. He works closely with local GPs, his team, social services and the Alzheimer's Society to achieve this. He also has a special interest in the use of cognitive behavioural psychotherapy (CBT) and mindfulness in older adults. He contributes to strategy work both nationally as an executive member of the Royal College of Psychiatrists Old Age Psychiatry faculty, and locally.

Chapter 1

How do you want your dementia to be?

Summary

- As the world's population ages, dementia is becoming much more common. This is the catch in us living longer lives.

- The rising incidence of dementia is a success story, mirroring the rise in the average human lifespan, and of humankind conquering infectious and contagious disease.

- The increasing possibility that many of us will develop dementia in the latter stages of life should prompt us to contemplate what our experience of dementia may be.

- Whilst it is known that memory and function decline in dementia, individual experiences of dementia are varied and not uniform tales of decay.

- Rather than ignoring the issue, we should think ahead about how we might cope with dementia if it should happen to us.

- Any of us may also find ourselves suddenly in the position of a carer for someone with dementia. It is sensible to consider what this might mean to us and what would be the most important issues if this arises.

I. (NOEL)

The UK and the world's population is ageing. By 2032, the number of people over 65 is projected to rise to around a quarter of the population.[1] Historically, the dramatic decline in births has been the main driver of population ageing in the UK and the rest of the developed world. More recently, a reduction in mortality and increased life expectancy have contributed to population ageing,[1] and in recent decades, improvement in mortality rates for older adults, rather than infants, has contributed most to improved life expectancies.[2] A consequence of increasing life expectancy has been a dramatic rise in the 'oldest old', the over-85 age group. It is the fastest growing demographic group in the UK and by 2032, the oldest old is expected to double to over three million people.[1]

The biggest risk factor for dementia is age. So, as the population ages, the prevalence of dementia will naturally increase. Globally, the expected numbers of people living with dementia are predicted nearly to double every 20 years and by 2030, over 65 million people will have dementia worldwide.[3] In the UK, it is predicted that by 2025 over a million people will be living with dementia.[4] But this is not an epidemic of dementia. The rising incidence of dementia is a success story, as noted in the recent review of risk factors by NIHR,[5] mirroring the rise in the average human lifespan and of humankind conquering infectious and contagious disease. A hundred years ago we would not have needed to contemplate dementia as it affected only a few fortunate enough to reach old age. Now the probability is that we will all face it – either our own or the care of someone close to us. This is the catch in us living longer lives.

Although we know that more people will be living with dementia, dementia prevalence figures don't tell us what the lives of people with dementia (PwD) will be like. At present, we know relatively little about the lives of people *currently* living with dementia. Although the epidemiology, pathology and biomedical aspects of the disease are well documented, the experiences of those living with conditions like dementia have, until now, been relatively absent in scientific and public discourse. Most media coverage of dementia is pervasively negative. However, whilst it is known that memory and function decline in dementia, quality of life is more complex and does not simply decline in line with loss of memory and function.[6] Individual experiences of dementia are varied and not uniform tales of decay. The rising prevalence of the condition, and the possibility that many of us will develop it in the latter stages of life, should prompt us to contemplate what our experience of dementia might be like. Is it purely a result of biological changes in the brain? How important are social factors? What can I do to improve the experience of dementia? How would I want my dementia to be? These questions are usually avoided earlier in life, but if they are considered now may make a big difference later.

II. (MARY)
Planning for dementia

Planning for dementia is rather less popular than planning for end of life. A few people have the foresight to draw up a lasting power of attorney (LPA) on a 'just in case' basis – perhaps rather more now than in the past – but the most common 'planning' that anyone does is limited to a plea to their families not to 'put me in a home' (see Chapter 8, page 167, for a discussion about the reluctance to go into residential care). Behind this lack of thought and planning lie many emotions. In my work, I frequently come across people who refuse to seek help and indeed, actively reject help offered to them. I meet people with elderly parents who are frustrated and angry at their parents' refusal to accept the possibility that they need any intervention. I meet the elderly themselves, who vigorously deny any need and who resent the well-meaning attempts of their children to 'interfere'. I work with care professionals who want to put measures in place for their clients that they believe will make their lives easier, or reduce risks to health and safety, but whose attempts to help are firmly rejected. I think that at the root of this reluctance lie some very deep fears – a fear of losing independence, a fear of losing control and a fear of being forced into a mode of life which has not been self-chosen.

A diagnosis of dementia does indeed mean a loss of independence and perhaps also a loss of self-control. People with dementia are unable to live independently, and one of the chief symptoms of the disease is the loss of the ability to control one's thoughts and actions. However, does the diagnosis need to lead to people being forced into a mode of life which they would not choose? One of the most memorable things I recall from working together with Noel was how often he used to attempt to explain to those diagnosed that if a person had a diagnosis but was well supported, in otherwise good health, and accepting of appropriate help, he or she could nevertheless lead a happy and fulfilled life. Each time I heard him explain this I would feel hopeful and yet apprehensive. The words were truly spoken but so few would (or perhaps could) take proper account of them.

In my experience people who are diagnosed seem to dismiss the explanation. They would assure us that they were quite able to manage their lives, that they were well supported (if they should need support), and that they would indeed accept appropriate help and support *when the time came*. No one ever seemed to think that the time for help and support was *now*. Carers accompanying the person diagnosed were more cautious. They usually understood that support was needed, but most often (except in cases of very late diagnosis) felt that they could offer what was needed. As a general rule, it seems to me that at the point of diagnosis most people do not have a real understanding of what the diagnosis means for the future. If this is the case with people who have a diagnosis and therefore already have some experience of the difficulties arising, how much harder must it be for those of us with full cognitive abilities to picture a future where we can no longer plan for the future, make planned and considered decisions, remember a recent experience or even understand what is going on around us? Yet this is the future we must picture if we want to live happy and fulfilled lives with dementia.

Issues to consider

Think about it now; think about how you want your dementia to be. It isn't enough to assume that if you have dementia you will no longer care about what happens to you. Research and empirical evidence show us that PwD do care – many care very deeply – about what happens in their lives. Many of the behavioural and psychological symptoms of dementia (BPSD) arise because PwD are unable to take action to alleviate their cares, or often to express their concerns even to those who are nearest to them. But now, at this moment, you are able to think about the future; you are able to consider what is important to you and you are able (and this can be so difficult) to think about how your life might be when those important things are swept away from you.

1. **Financial and legal planning.** Some things are easier to consider than others. Many of us are able to picture the possibility that we may be unable to manage our financial affairs at some point in our lives. Arranging a lasting power of attorney (LPA) – that is, giving someone we trust the power to manage our money and property if we should be unable to do this – is a sensible option and many people who

will make no other arrangements for the future feel able to do this. But if you really want to retain control of how your dementia will be, you need to go further than this.

2. **Writing a 'dementia plan'.** Consider what makes your life 'worth living' and discuss it with your family. Is it your work, your business, your hobbies, your family, your friends, your ability to hear music, to read, to walk out alone, to work in the garden, to travel, to choose what and when to eat? As dementia progresses you may lose the ability to enjoy any or all of these. What then? You could write a 'dementia plan' which covers all these points and lodge it along with your will, your LPA and your advance decision statement (you have drawn up all these, of course!), and this might appear a sensible option. It would be a dreary exercise though, and in the event, it might not apply as much as you might think. Many of us consider how we might feel in a certain situation – if we were to lose the ability to walk perhaps, due to accident or illness, or if we were confronted by the need for some unpleasant medical treatment such as chemotherapy – and give thought to what our plans and decisions might be, but until confronted by that very situation it is impossible to know for certain what we might think, want and actually decide. Dementia is no different. Some people whom I meet just after diagnosis state that they have always believed a diagnosis of dementia to be a 'fate worse than death' but very few express a wish to hasten death in order to avoid it.

3. **Managing expectations.** Noel and I have some differences of opinion about how happy PwD actually are (see Chapter 3, page 43), but we both agree that many people living with the diagnosis have a good quality of life, and indeed express this fact to us verbally during clinic consultations. The truth is that expectations change as cognitive abilities deteriorate. When one can no longer pursue a 12-mile hike, one may still enjoy a

stroll around the local park. Those who can no longer follow the plot of a film may still enjoy watching a nature or travel programme on TV for the action and scenery. People who are no longer able to read a novel frequently enjoy reciting poetry or having it read to them. So, for example, a healthy and intelligent 80-year-old may view with horror the idea of spending time in a day centre taking part in the activities on offer there. Indeed, I have lost count of the carers who have told me categorically that the person they care for would never countenance this – always hated socialising, never joined clubs, disliked card or board games, hated quizzes, and would dislike the experience intensely. No doubt this is true of the person who used to be – the person the carer used to know. However, someone who is no longer able to understand a U3A lecture, read a book or a newspaper, or follow a radio or TV programme may be glad to be included in a group solving a crossword together, or may enjoy being able to chat to others over a drink without feeling they have to strain to follow a conversation, may just enjoy cheerful company and surroundings other than those they see every day.

4. **Acknowledging key personality traits.** It may not be appropriate to write a 'dementia plan' in terms of what you want to happen in all the situations you might envisage, but there are likely to be some things which you may consider to be vitally important. On the many occasions when I have been involved with care homes, hospitals or day care centres in trying to establish why a person with dementia is expressing 'challenging behaviour', or BPSD, the final solution usually turns out not to be connected with a particular activity or personality clash with a care-giver or resident. The problem is usually due to a misunderstanding of a basic characteristic of the person we are trying to help. So, for example, some people really dislike a 'dead silence', and when they are left

alone in their room in the care home they become frightened and angry because it is so quiet. Conversely, others find constant noise unbearable and exhibit difficult behaviour when they are expected to sit in a communal lounge with the television on or with music playing. At day centres, we have often found that people who get anxious and restless simply need to be allowed to go outside in the garden as and when they choose – many people dislike the idea of being 'shut in'. (I fulminate elsewhere in this book on the many care homes where 'going outside' is considered an activity only to be allowed on warm sunny days with the express permission of the team manager on duty, see page 170). There are people who cannot bear to sit in an untidy room and others who intensely dislike someone 'clearing up' around them. It is these more fundamental things, which are worth pinpointing when you consider how you would like your dementia to be. What sort of things would make life unbearable to you? And what sort of things would ultimately make you feel that life was worth living?

5. **Understanding the implications of becoming a carer.** You should also consider the possibility of a future affected by dementia as a caregiver. What will you do if your life partner is diagnosed with dementia? Or if your parent (or even perhaps your child) receives a diagnosis? Your own life will be changed by the diagnosis. How do you think you might cope? With the best will in the world – and many people do have the will and the determination to look after someone they love as long as they can – your manner of life will not be the same as you might have envisaged. Your peace of mind, your time and your own health may all be affected. In many ways, it can be harder to imagine life as a caregiver than life as a person with dementia. I know this. I discuss in later chapters the many cases where caregivers reject help at the

point of diagnosis because they are unable to picture a time when things will be so much more difficult than they are now. It doesn't matter how carefully the consultant explains the prognosis or how often I describe the progressive nature of the illness, the human brain seems to find it difficult to absorb the reality of something it has not yet experienced. But considering what life might be like as a carer, and giving thought to the things that are important to you, may be wise.

It is easy to become absorbed in being a carer, to gradually sublimate yourself to the needs of another, to allow your own interests to take second place, to be always 'on duty', to be constantly watchful for the needs and risks that arise, and to slowly, very slowly lose your social contacts, your companions and your family relationships as you become more and more absorbed into your caring role. That is a depressing suggestion, and in fact you may shy away from even considering the possibility of this happening to you. Still, this is another thing that you should think about, discuss with other family members and even plan for.

REFERENCES

1. Dunnell K. Ageing and mortality in the UK. *Population Trends* 2008; 134: 6-23.

2. Christensen K, Doblhammer G, Rau R, et al. Ageing populations: the challenges ahead. *The Lancet* 2009; 374(9696): 1196-208.

3. Prince M, Bryce R, Albanese E, Wimon A, Ribeiro W, Ferri CP. The global prevalence of dementia: A systematic review and metaanalysis. *Alzheimer's & Dementia: The Journal of the Alzheimer's Association* 2013; 9(1): 63-75.

4. Prince M, Knapp M, Guerchet M, McCrone P, Prina M, Comas-Herrera A, Wittenberg R, Adelaja B, King D. *Dementia UK: Update.* London: Alzheimer's Society; 2014.

5. Livingston G, Sommerlad A, Orgeta V et al. Dementia prevention, intervention, and care. *The Lancet*. 2017 Jul 19. doi: 10.1016/S0140-6736(17)31363-6.

6. Banerjee S, Smith SC, Lamping DL, Harwood RH, Foley B, Smith P, Murray J, Prince M, Levin E, Mann A, Knapp M. Quality of life in dementia: more than just cognition. An analysis of associations with quality of life in dementia. *Journal of Neurology, Neurosurgery & Psychiatry* 2006; 77(2): 146-48.

Chapter 2

The limits of the medical model in dementia

Summary

- Current medical understandings of dementia focus on pathology and deficit.

- The concept of dementia continues to evolve.

- The increasing prevalence of dementia is a natural consequence of the increasing human lifespan.

- There is a wide overlap of normal and abnormal between late-onset dementia and normal ageing.

- Currently, there is no definitive test that 'proves' a diagnosis of dementia. The diagnosis is made on the results of cognitive testing, a history of decline in function and collaborative information from near relatives/close companions.

- The difference between dementia and mild cognitive impairment is not precise.

- A diagnosis of dementia can be helpful in opening up support pathways to people who are struggling to cope. However, it can also be demoralising and stigmatising.

- Cognitive enhancers are not 'miracle medicines' and give only limited help to a small number of patients.

- Although there is no cure for dementia, improving care will alleviate much distress and fear associated with the condition.

- Good support and information can make a difference to how people cope with the diagnosis.

I. (NOEL)
The current (medical) paradigm of dementia

The prevalent Western understanding of 'dementia' in 2017 remains primarily that it is the result of a collection of degenerative brain diseases that are best explained by corresponding cellular level changes in the brain. These include:

- **Alzheimer's disease**, often thought to be the most common type of dementia. It usually presents with a disturbance of short-term memory, and is associated with the collection of abnormal protein, called B-amyloid, in the brain in the form of plaques and tangles. The role of abnormal production of β-amyloid as the cause (and potential treatment) of Alzheimer's disease is called the amyloid-hypothesis.

- **Vascular dementia** typically presents with patchy executive deficits: a slowing of mental processes and a 'stepwise' pattern of decline, where deterioration can occur dramatically then plateau, in contrast to the gradual decline of Alzheimer's. This decline is thought to be due to the death of brain cells due to progressive damage to blood vessels and blood flow within the brain.

- **Lewy body dementia**, like Parkinson's dementia, is thought to be due to the accumulation of abnormal brain deposits, called Lewy bodies, in the brain and is associated with a fluctuating progression, visual hallucinations and movement difficulties, as seen in Parkinson's disease.

- **Parkinson's dementia** is a dementia where progressive cognitive impairment typically develops after the onset of the motor symptoms of Parkinson's disease.

- **'Mixed dementia'** syndromes occur where there is an overlap of two syndromes, typically Alzheimer's disease and vascular dementia, and is considered by some to be the most common 'type' of dementia.

- **Fronto-temporal dementias (FTDs)** are a loose collection of atypical dementia syndromes, which typically occur at a younger age and can affect language and behaviour more than memory.

However, this list of types of dementia is constantly evolving, as we shall see later in this chapter.

Diagnosing dementia

It is often a surprise to people undergoing a memory test that, even in 2017, dementia is a 'clinical diagnosis'. This means the diagnosis is largely made on the person's history and through cognitive testing rather than being confirmed by a diagnostic test, such as a scan or histology (the collection and microscopic examination of brain cells which remains rather impractical during life). Dementia is diagnosed on the basis of clinical criteria, such as:

- Progressive impairment in cognitive functions such as

memory, language or 'executive skills' (such as problem solving or multi-tasking) that are severe enough to affect daily function.

- Non-cognitive or so-called 'behavioural and psychological symptoms of dementia' (BPSD) that also occur as the dementia progresses.

- Elimination of other causes – that is, whether the impairment can be explained by any reversible medical or psychiatric cause, such as thyroid disease, other brain disease such as delirium or psychiatric illness such as depression or anxiety. A 'dementia screen', which typically involves blood tests and sometimes a brain scan prior to referral to a memory specialist, is a confusing term here as it is actually a screen for other causes of memory loss, rather than dementia.

- Whether or not the presenting cognitive symptoms are of a degree to affect function. If they are, then a 'mild cognitive impairment' (MCI) can be 'diagnosed'. However, this remains a very problematic diagnosis as the boundary between MCI and early dementia has shifted over time, as the definition of daily function has changed. Twenty years ago, function was defined in very basic terms such as being able to dress and feed oneself, whilst nowadays it is defined in more instrumental terms, such as being able to manage one's finances, use transport, or technology such as the telephone. The practice of dividing patients into MCI and dementia groups also has a number of other consequences, which will be discussed in Chapter 8 (page 162).

- Whether the symptoms are consistent with young-onset or later-onset (or senile) dementias. Young-onset dementias are defined, rather arbitrarily, as those occurring before 65 years of age, and despite being grouped under the same dementia term, are usually very different from later-onset dementias in respect to their onset, cause, presentation and prognosis. In senile dementias, the degree of overlap between normal ageing and later-onset dementias can also be problematic and will be discussed later.

The evolving concept of dementia

Dementia has always been a difficult, slippery and problematic word. It is currently defined in the Merriam-Webster dictionary 'as a serious mental disorder that prevents one from living a safe and normal life'.[1] The contextual sentence used to illustrate the meaning is 'doctors were able to treat the patient's dementia with drugs and thus allow him to function on his own'.[1]

However, the word 'dementia' has not always had such a medical meaning. The condition has been observed for at least 2000 years and 'dementia' has remained a mercurial term, changing meaning according to the predominant thinking of the time. Ancient physicians and philosophers such as Aristotle and Galen considered dementia to be an inevitable consequence of ageing. They normalised the onset of senile dementia and considered ageing itself as the disease.

However, at other times over history, dementia has been viewed as madness, possession or even a consequence of sinning. The medical model of dementia as an illness really took hold towards the end of the 17th century with physicians such as William Cullen viewing dementia as a clinical syndrome that could be observed, diagnosed and classified. This biomedical model of dementia took even more hold following the publication of the work of Aloysius Alzheimer (1864–1915), who linked the illness of dementia with directly observable microscopic changes in the brain such as clumps and tangles of protein called senile plaques and neurofibrillary tangles, as well as changes in brain blood vessels.

Although medicine as a discipline has changed much since Auguste Deter's brain was examined by Alzheimer under a microscope in 1906, difficulties with the exact meaning of the word dementia persist. Kraeplin, a German psychiatrist and colleague of Alzheimer, used the term 'dementia' to refer to both schizophrenia (praecox) and late-onset neurodegeneration (senilis), and although the concept of Alzheimer's disease has become synonymous with dementia for most people, 'dementia' has also become an umbrella term for progressive memory disorders of any cause. As noted earlier, these include Alzheimer's disease, vascular dementia, Lewy body disease or dementia, Parkinson's disease dementia and fronto-temporal dementia.

Although these more specific dementia syndromes sound more precise and exact, they are conundrums in themselves. They can be difficult to diagnose precisely during life. An individual patient can also present with features of two or more different dementias leading to a diagnosis of 'mixed dementia' as mentioned already. And although certain brain scan findings are thought to be linked to specific conditions, such as shrinkage in certain parts of the brain in Alzheimer's and signs of blood vessel damage in vascular dementia, the radiological diagnosis (made on scan findings) does not always match the clinical diagnosis in the person.

Another problem with dementia diagnoses is that the way they are made has changed over time. The inclusion of vascular (or blood vessel) changes within the definition of Alzheimer's disease has, for example, changed over the last 100 years. Initially, the presence of vascular changes was accepted as part of Alzheimer's disease, then as an exclusion criterion (to suggest vascular dementia instead), and more recently included again in a diagnosis of 'dementia in Alzheimer's, atypical or mixed type'.

This ongoing instability in defining dementia syndromes and the confusion in their naming is reflected in how dementia is conceptualised in current diagnostic guidelines used by psychiatrists. An example is the *ICD-10 Classification of Mental and Behavioural Disorders*,[2] which defines and categorises dementia. Here, dementia is divided into Alzheimer's disease, vascular dementia and 'dementia in other diseases classified elsewhere' (which includes Picks' disease and dementia in Parkinson's disease). These are further divided into additional sub-categories based on onset and other clinical features.

This can give the false impression that these categories are discrete and mutually exclusive disease entities, belying the fact that patients often present with symptom mixtures from several dementia categories. 'Mixed type dementia', however, is buried within a sub-code of Alzheimer's disease, despite increasing evidence that this may be the most common dementia type, particularly for older patients.[3] Lewy body dementia, which may be the second most common form of dementia by some estimates,[4] is not even listed in *ICD-10*. Instead, doctors need to use 'dementia in Parkinson's disease' when clinically coding. Although Lewy body and Parkinson's dementia are related, they are not the same. Cognitive impairment within Parkinson's disease is complex and can be due to medications and not progress into a dementia.[5] Hence the attempt to divide dementia into categories, using systems like *ICD-10*, can create more confusion that it solves.

Another example of the unstable concept of dementia, both in terms of the valid application of these diagnoses to patients in life and in the instability of the terminology itself, is 'fronto-temporal dementia' (FTD). This umbrella term refers to dementia that preferentially affects the frontal and temporal lobes of the brain. This results in different clinical syndromes, which can vary significantly from Alzheimer's and other forms of dementia, usually affecting language or behaviour well before memory.

Currently the FTD umbrella term includes semantic dementia, progressive aphasia and 'behavioural variant fronto-temporal dementia' (bvFTD).

Confusingly, the term FTD itself is missing from *ICD-10* and instead the archetypal form of FTD, Pick's disease, is used instead. Pick's disease and FTD are often used interchangeably by clinicians, but bvFTD is often the implied meaning. To further confuse matters, clinical consensus criteria used to diagnose 'bvFTD' changes regularly, having been revised four times in the last 20 years. The reality of the dynamic FTD concept is that it remains unstable with regard to its meaning to clinicians. What does it include? What doesn't it include? And that is before we begin a discussion of what the diagnosis means to people affected by the condition(s) who are younger, and who usually experience a delay in diagnosis due to the atypical nature of the presentation.

It is not entirely certain how long the term 'dementia' will persist given the current trend in medicine for reductionism and more 'precise' diagnoses. Survival of the word may depend on which medical specialty continues to 'own' dementia. Currently in the United Kingdom, psychiatrists are the main specialists who diagnose and treat dementia in partnership with general practitioners. Psychiatrists are a mixed bunch, with some believing in categorical diagnoses more readily than others. Neurologists, as per their training, are usually more inclined to give more precise diagnostic labels, whilst GPs and geriatricians often apply more descriptive terms with their patients, such as 'cognitive impairment'. The latter term is perhaps less stigmatising, but also vague.

The two disciplines of neurology and psychiatry may coalesce at some time in the next 100 years as the secrets of the brain are unlocked and the divide between behaviour and biology is narrowed. If the neurology paradigm dominates in this new union, then the umbrella term of 'dementia' may become obsolete and instead be devolved into specific, more biologically based dementia syndromes. However, given that 'dementia' has somehow survived as a clinical term this long, it may well be that we are stuck with it. Perhaps, through more frequent usage as our population ages, 'dementia' will assume a more benign meaning.

Why does the medical model currently prevail in dementia?

The theory that dementia can be attributed to a clear cause, such as the accumulation of abnormal amyloid, Lewy bodies or abnormal blood vessels in the brain, is attractive. If the mercurial, bewildering symptoms of cognitive and behavioural disturbances in dementia can be linked to a clear, observable change in the field of a microscope, then this has an attractive coherence for everyone – patients, carers and doctors. You have 'x' in your brain, so this is why you think 'y' and feel 'z'. Medicine as a whole relies on this kind of reasoning, whereby complex phenomena can be explained and reduced, usually by a medical 'expert', using an underlying simple explanatory theory. This reductionism has been the historic source of the mythology of medicine. Jenner performed the first vaccination in 1796 against serious infectious disease, observing that dairy maids infected with cowpox were immune against the more virulent small pox. John Snow arrested the spread of a dysentery epidemic in London in 1854 by discovering that cholera was spread in water, and removed the handles of a public water pump in Broad Street.

More recently, in 1982 Barry Marshall and Robin Warren discovered that the bacterium *Helicobacter pylori* is the cause of most stomach ulcers, and that antibiotics combined with antacids could cure these without recourse to surgery.

Even where a definitive cure has been elusive, a reductionist approach in medicine has paid real dividends in managing other conditions such as AIDS. Through the isolation of the causative human immunodeficiency virus and the development of highly specific and effective anti-retroviral treatment, AIDS has evolved over the last three decades from a fatal disease viewed as a plague to a more chronic disease, like diabetes, that can be managed with appropriate medication. Given that biomedical science has succeeded in curing and managing so many illnesses, the idea that dementia can be similarly cured has an irresistible allure. Surely all that is needed with dementia is more research, more time, and more money? Surely a cure must just be around the corner? And then catastrophic predictions of a dementia tsunami, and of impossible demand on stretched health and social care systems, can be ignored.

The wide overlap between normal and abnormal in later-onset dementia

Distinguishing normal from abnormal in an organ as complex as the brain is not a simple task. This is partly because the normal ageing brain is not always easy to define. Carol Brayne rightly points out that in any discussion of dementia and cognitive health, ageing is the proverbial elephant in the room.[6] This is because the definition of a healthy ageing brain is not universally agreed, which makes any subsequent discussion of the unhealthy brain inherently difficult.[6] This concept also challenges the positivist and mainstream view of dementia as a disease that you either have or don't have.

Carol Brayne writes extensively regarding the overlap of disease and normal ageing in Alzheimer's disease. Most doctors and medical students, and many patients, would describe the pathognomonic signs of Alzheimer's disease (that is, the cellular changes seen in the brains of people with Alzheimer's at post mortem autopsy) as consisting of amyloid plaques and neurofibrillary tangles. However, these changes (as well as changes seen in blood vessels in vascular dementia) are often seen in older people without dementia.[6] Equally, a significant minority of people in later life who have severe Alzheimer's disease do not seem to have amyloid plaques in their brains. This latter group in particular challenges the amyloid hypothesis and the idea that the underlying biology is always the defining pathognomonic factor in dementia.[6]

It is also important to remember that Alzheimer first described the classic cellular changes associated with his disease in the brain of a 58-year-old. As in most diseases, the earlier the age of onset of dementia, the stronger the correlation with physical and observable changes in the brain. Although the genetics, presentation and prognosis of young-onset dementias are different when compared with older-onset (or so-called senile) dementias, there is often a conflation of the two. The assumption that senile-onset and young-onset dementias share the same clear cellular basis is widespread. However, the pathway to older adult dementia is more varied and dependent on other individual and environmental factors. Carol Brayne reminds us that the notion of the solitary illness is a fallacy for most older people with the condition.[6]

Dementia for most people in later life is the result of a complex interplay of cognitive resilience and vulnerabilities, played out over the lifespan. Given that the global rise in dementia is occurring mostly in older people, this means that dementia is becoming more heterogeneous and more difficult to define as clear categorical illnesses, such Alzheimer's disease or vascular dementia, resulting from amyloid plaques and vascular changes respectively. This also means that the search for the 'magic bullet', or cure, for dementia is likely to be fruitless. This is because when we talk about a cure for dementia, we are actually talking about a cure for past stressors over the lifespan and ageing in the majority of cases.

Benefits of the biomedical model of dementia

What are the benefits of a traditional biomedical approach in dementia? Although I have criticised reductionist thinking in relation to dementia above, there have been clear benefits from this approach. The redefining of it as a disease, rather than as an inevitable senile phase of late life, has led to a new optimism in an area traditionally untouched by medicine. Diagnosis is now seen as the first step in obtaining initial help for people with dementia (PwD). This has led to the development and expansion of the memory clinics model where people with suspected cognitive impairment are referred for assessment for likelihood of dementia. Further investigations to confirm a diagnosis can occur and individualised post-diagnostic advice in relation to further care and crisis planning can be given. My experience of working with staff in memory services has been universally positive and they are a multidisciplinary group of practitioners committed to helping PwD and their carers. Although the provision of post-diagnostic support varies by location, it is clear that many PwD and their carers now benefit from excellent individual and group support that was completely absent 20 years ago.

This biomedical focus has also driven improvements in the understanding of the condition and led to the development of evidence-based practice for patients with dementia along the whole 'care pathway' from diagnosis to death. The development of cognitive enhancers, for example, has resulted in the first effective treatments that can slow the progression of cognitive decline in dementia. Other research has examined numerous aspects of dementia, such as the natural progression of the condition(s), its relationship with other conditions and the use of medication and other approaches that can help those with behavioural and psychological symptoms of dementia. There is also increasing research activity looking at whether scans and other tests can help in diagnosing dementia sooner, or in fact prevent the development of the condition in susceptible individuals.

How can the biomedical model fail people with dementia?

Whilst a biomedical approach has led to improvements in the lives of PwD, it also has pitfalls. In particular, whether being diagnosed with dementia can do more harm than good. As we have seen, the word 'dementia' has been a source of fear since its inception, and in popular culture, is often a state feared more than death. Diagnosing dementia is a complex transaction between doctor and patient, not just because of the inherent difficulties in making a clinical diagnosis but also because of the varied meanings associated with the word. Dementia is often received as a feared and unwanted label by patients and their family, terrifying and perplexing in equal measure, rather than a benign clinical term attached by doctors to the difficulties they are having.

In her book *Illness as a Metaphor*, Susan Sontag describes this harmful process of diagnosis with cancer, rather than dementia, but her perspectives provide insights relevant to both conditions. She says that 'as long as a particular disease is treated as an evil, invisible predator, not just a disease, most people … will indeed be demoralised by learning what disease they have.'[7] She also points out that doctors are also heavily influenced by the meanings they associate with a particular illness and this affects the candour with which a diagnosis is given.[7] This may account for the hesitancy of many doctors to diagnose dementia because of their feelings of therapeutic impotence and failure. It can also represent an unconscious collusion with a broader societal expectation that living with the dementia must be a universally negative experience, associated with relentless daily decline and eventual disintegration.

Mary and I have certainly witnessed the attempts of families of patients presenting with dementia to protect them from the diagnosis, using more acceptable terms such as 'cognitive impairment' or 'memory loss' rather than the D-word. We have, at times, been knowingly guilty of this collusion, when we felt that diagnosing dementia in explicit terms would cause distress or more harm than good.

A biomedical focus in dementia also carries other limitations, beyond the process of diagnosis. In particular, it can disempower families and carers who feel they are helpless in the face of a biological curse like dementia. Dementia can also assume a master status in the minds of carers, degrading care through the loss of personhood and the process of 'othering' whereby carers only see dementia rather than the person.[8,9] This is discussed in Chapter 4 (page 54).

The mirage of cure

The biomedical model dominates contemporary narratives around dementia in the popular media. Headlines frequently herald a single miracle cure for the epidemic of dementia as being just around the corner. However, a cure like this seems unlikely for most PwD, given that it is not a single disease, and that there is an increasing overlap between 'normal' and 'abnormal' development in the brain as we age.[6] This mirage of cure also has a number of negative consequences, including creating false expectations of what modern medicine can achieve and displacing more important narratives around dementia about ageing, death, care and the role of society.

As modern medicine appears to progress on multiple fronts each year, people's expectations of what it can offer dementia appear to increase also. However, it needs to be remembered there are no precedents of any degenerative neurological condition ever being 'cured'. Families sometimes seem to forget that we remain mortal. In our memory clinic work together, Mary and I are often surprised about the level of family expectation about the role of medicine in helping a person with dementia. We frequently have to manage expectations about the use of medications in dementia, sometimes for people in extreme old age. In particular, we have to explain that cognitive enhancers such as donepezil and memantine are not miracle drugs, and can often cause more harm than good. And although other antidepressant or antipsychotic drugs can certainly be helpful in certain cases, non-pharmacological approaches for the distressed, depressed, anxious or paranoid person with dementia should always be the first port of call.

People attending our clinic are often surprised when I explain that the evidence base for the use of medication, such as antidepressants for depression, is poor in dementia.[10] They are similarly disappointed that, despite an increase in biomedical research into dementia, and a number of trials involving unpronounceable new drugs, such as bapineuzumab, there is no indication that any of these will be a panacea for the majority of people with memory problems or dementia. There have been many false dawns in the search for the elusive cure, such as vaccines against amyloid proteins, which appear ineffective and potentially harmful.[11,12]

I often find it more rewarding in my memory clinic to steer the conversation away from the biomedical ground of diagnosis and medication to sociological territory, such as discussion of the individual, the process of ageing and care, death and the broader contexts of politics and society. I explain that although it is my role to examine evidence to support and apply a diagnosis of dementia, I increasingly feel this is only part of my work. Mary has borne witness to the increasing sociological emphasis in my post-diagnostic discussion, and that I often emphasise a number of points with individual patients. Namely, that memory problems and dementia are a natural consequence of ageing and increasing life span. And that although more people now survive diseases such as cancers, strokes and heart attacks, a final wave of challenges present themselves in the form of cognitive impairments, dementias and frailty.

To make the point less abstractly, memory clinics 100 or 200 years ago would have had considerably less trade, as few people survived infectious and other diseases to develop any concerns with their memory. I also like to quote the statistic that a third of babies born in 2015 will live long enough to develop a memory problem such as dementia,[13] and as a consequence future memory clinic colleagues will be very busy! It is important to contextualise these comments carefully to ensure that they are not interpreted as being facetious, but rather an epidemiological framing of the individual.

Similarly, although discussions of mortality and death must be explored sensitively, they can be very helpful in contextualising an individual's presentation of dementia and, in particular, neutralising the 'rhetoric of loss' that can occur on diagnosis. 'Rhetoric of loss' implies a preoccupation with an idealised past rather than the present, and was first described in relation to idealised descriptions of past life in William Faulkner's novels.[14] More times than not, I find that using sociological understandings of dementia alongside biomedical ones helps wrestle the narrative of dementia away from being purely a pathological state, towards a more positive manifestation of us living longer lives. This can then be the first shift towards PwD viewing themselves as successful survivors in life, rather than passive victims of a medical condition.

II. (MARY)
Avoiding dementia

This may be a good moment to consider what we can do to avoid dementia in our later years. I have discussed this in other books in more detail,[15] and we do know that certain 'risk factors' raise the likelihood of a future diagnosis of dementia, and that many of these risks can be addressed. The time to consider reducing these risks is now. This is one of the key messages in the NHIR report on Risk Factors for Dementia published in July 2017.[16]

- **Regular exercise** benefits the body and the mind. People are often surprised to discover that physical exercise is more beneficial to the mind then so-called 'brain exercise', but there is ample evidence to support this,[15] and the same evidence shows that regular moderate exercise is the key – you don't have to be a marathon runner to reap the benefit. Walking, gardening and leisure activities like non-competitive cycling, bowls, dancing and swimming, all count as exercise. It is, of course, important to keep using your brain but in this respect what we should be thinking about is helping the brain form new connections.

- **Doing new things**. Crosswords and puzzles are pleasant ways for some people to pass the time but they are unlikely to develop new connections in your brain, especially if you always choose to do the ones in your regular daily paper. Your brain is strengthened and developed by new experiences and new activities. Learning a new language, learning to play a musical instrument, trying a new hobby, going to new places, reading about a subject you don't usually bother with, are all ways to develop brain connections and keep your brain active.

- **Social interaction.** Another factor known to be significant is the continued connections we make with other people. Those who are 'loners' and who avoid mixing are at a higher risk of developing dementia. As we grow older there is a continuous temptation to 'stick with what we know', to avoid new experiences, to mix with old friends and make fewer attempts to meet new. It is more difficult to form new networks as the society we move in becomes more restricted. But age and infirmity are no longer a good excuse to live in a restricted manner. Technology has benefits as well as disadvantages and it is easier than ever before to make new contacts and to learn new things, thanks to mobile communication devices, the internet, and the many forms of media now available.

- **Diet.** Nutrition is important if we want to avoid dementia, and there is increasing evidence to show that the diet suitable for adults in mid-life may not be the best for older people who want to keep fit, active and mentally alert. In particular low-fat foods are not suitable for older people as a general rule (and should not be routinely eaten by people who actually have dementia).

- **Other conditions.** Some physical illnesses are known to increase the risk factor for dementia – in particular, type 2 (maturity-onset) diabetes is a very high risk factor, as well as a dangerous disease in its own right. Current medical opinion seems to suggest that most of us can avoid developing maturity-onset diabetes by following sensible lifestyle options.

Using the diagnosis alongside the person

As I follow up with people who have been diagnosed, and with their carers, it can be salutary to realise that the explanations given in the diagnostic clinic are often neither remembered nor understood. At some stage, most carers will telephone me to say that the person they care for is 'getting worse' and it is time to see Noel again to talk about increasing the medication. The general belief seems to be that it really is all a question of medication. Like other chronic conditions (diabetes, multiple sclerosis) the impression is that the disease can be continually 'managed' with an increase or change of medication. In our clinic, Noel has always been careful to explain that memory drugs are not wonder drugs, and that the efficacy varies from person to person. Still, carers often ask me why the person they care for does not seem to be any better or 'when will the drug kick in?'

In Western society, there is a deeply held impression that medical science has pretty well found a cure or a treatment for everything (the excepted disease is cancer, but as the media and fund-raising campaign literature keep assuring us 'it is only a matter of time'). It may be that the constant publicity attendant upon 'finding a cure' prevents society in general from understanding and accepting dementia as a disability, which will not get better. As a psychologist said to me once, 'You can retrain a brain but you need a brain to train.' Some well-publicised 'therapies' such as 'Rementia'[17] avoid this uncomfortable truth.

The medical model of dementia may have little to offer in the present day, and this can make difficulties for doctors who are expected by their patients to offer the right cure or treatment. My position as a dementia support worker has always involved supporting and advising PwD and their carers about their care options, as well as sometimes helping people to understand the diagnosis, and the benefits and limitations of medical treatment. The single most beneficial advance for PwD and their carers has come from the closer collaboration (in our local area at least) between the Community Mental Health Team (the diagnostic element), the GPs (who are gate-keepers to other services) and the service that dementia support workers offer. Carers have frequently praised 'our joined-up service' and PwD have told me that they value my presence in the clinic as someone who knows them well and works closely with the doctor.

Another problem arises with the wish for a specific diagnosis. As Noel points out above, the diagnosis is a slippery customer – people can show signs indicative of more than one form of dementia and symptoms can change as the disease progresses. Eyesight problems, for example, can manifest themselves very early – I had one client who spent six months having his sight investigated before he was diagnosed – or much later in the progress of the disease. It is not always understood that sight problems can be a symptom in up to 70 per cent of cases. Carers who use the internet to gain information and yet do not realise this, may state that the person they care for has Lewy body disease 'because they have trouble with their vision'.

Is early diagnosis beneficial?

There is a drive for earlier diagnosis and in some cases I question the benefit of this. Early diagnosis is helpful if it makes a difference to the progress of a disease or indeed (as in some cancers) means that a cure is more likely. Neither is true for dementia. True, many PwD will benefit from earlier diagnosis if there is good post-diagnostic support, but this is not always the case. Carers especially may, if they follow advice, find that support in the early stages results in less stress overall. Memory drugs can help some people to have an enhanced quality of life for a few months, but there is no 'magic window' of opportunity when these drugs must be given. Sometimes early diagnosis can have a dramatically detrimental effect. Often clients have told me that their friends treat them differently once the diagnosis becomes known. Some people have had travel insurance refused upon diagnosis. The biggest fear (and one which stops many from consulting their doctor) is that they will be stopped from driving.

Frequently people will reject support in the first weeks after diagnosis and this is their absolute right. Sometimes this is the result of a failure to understand the diagnosis correctly, sometimes because of a belief that the disease will not progress and that although there are deficiencies 'we can cope'. I believe that often people avoid following up offers of support due to shock following the diagnosis. A diagnosis of dementia can equate in the mind of some people to a diagnosis of disaster and the reaction is shock and disbelief. I find it strange that very few people are offered any kind of post-diagnostic support through the statutory medical services. The dementia support service of the Alzheimer's Society does offer this post-diagnostic support, but it is most often accepted when suggested by a doctor. There is an interesting, and perhaps natural, resistance to any approach made from an independent service, but a recommendation from 'the doctor' is generally acceptable. In our area, the close collaboration between the Community Mental Health Team and our service means that more people receive support after diagnosis, and in my experience, this results in a longer period of 'coping', including less carer stress and, particularly, in the PwD feeling that their feelings and emotions are being addressed.

I believe that the medical model of dementia, which sees dementia as 'a clinical syndrome characterised by global cognitive impairment representing a decline from a previous level of functioning', is not helpful to those diagnosed, or to the people who care for them. It may be that the so-called 'social model' of dementia, which seeks to understand the emotions and behaviours of the PwD by placing him or her within the context of his or her social circumstances and biography, also has its limitations. We might perhaps consider instead the 'natural model of dementia', which understands dementia as a consequence of survival of many other perils (including, as suggested previously, infectious disease, heart disease, cancer and mental life traumas of all kinds), and indicates a strength rather than a weakness, an indication of survival rather than a prediction of a disastrous end.

Things to consider after a diagnosis

1. Understand your diagnosis – get information from a reliable source – even if you can't face reading it all now you may want to later.

2. Address important practical considerations such as drawing up an LPA (lasting power of attorney) and informing the DVLA (the driving licence authority for those in the UK) of the diagnosis. Talk to your family about advance care directives.

3. Find out about local support organisations and activities.

4. Think about and discuss future lifestyle decisions that may arise. For example, consider the risks and benefits of living at home or moving to residential care.

5. Start to think about the people you want around you to manage risk and potential future difficulties. Talk to your relatives about these issues so they know what to do if they need to make these decisions on your behalf.

6. Don't be afraid to tell others about your memory problems and dementia. It is nothing to be ashamed of, and the more people talk about this openly the better.

7. Doctors may be the experts on medicine, but you are the expert on you. Ask your doctor lots of questions, particularly about your greatest fears. It is better that they are answered, rather than becoming a source of worry and rumination.

8. Educate your doctors. Tell them about your life and who you are. Make sure that your diagnosis does not become a label which defines you.

REFERENCES

1. Merriam-Webster Thesaurus. *Dementia*. http://www.merriamwebster.com/thesaurus/dementia (accessed 22 June 2017).

2. WHO. *ICD-10 Classification of Mental and Behavioural Disorders. Diagnostic Criteria for Research*. Geneva: WHO; 1993.

3. Neuropathology Group. Pathological correlates of late-onset dementia in a multicentre, community-based population in England and Wales. Neuropathology Group of the Medical Research Council Cognitive Function and Ageing Study (MRC CFAS). *The Lancet* 2001; 357(9251): 169.

4. McKeith I, Mintzer J, Aarsland D, et al. Dementia with Lewy bodies. *The Lancet Neurology* 2004; 3(1): 19-28.

5. Dilley M, Fleminger S. Advances in neuropsychiatry: clinical implications. *Advances in psychiatric treatment* 2006; 12(1): 23-34.

6. Brayne C. The elephant in the room – healthy brains in later life, epidemiology and public health. *Nature Reviews Neuroscience* 2007; 8(3): 233-39.

7. Sontag S. *Illness as metaphor and AIDS and its metaphors* London: Macmillan; 2001; page 7.

8. Doyle PJ, Rubinstein RL. Person-centered dementia care and the cultural matrix of othering. *The Gerontologist* 2014; 54(6): 952-63.

9. Touhy TA. Dementia, personhood, and nursing: Learning from a nursing situation. *Nursing Science Quarterly* 2004; 17(1): 43-49.

10. Bains J, Birks J, Dening T. *Antidepressants for treating depression in dementia*. The Cochrane Library; 2002.

11. Holmes C, Boche D, Wilkinson D, et al. Long-term effects of Aβ42 immunisation in Alzheimer's disease: follow-up of a randomised, placebo-controlled phase I trial. *The Lancet* 2008; 372(9634): 216-23.

12. Orgogozo J-M, Gilman S, Dartigues J-F, et al. Subacute meningoencephalitis in a subset of patients with AD after Aβ42 immunization. *Neurology* 2003; 61(1): 46-54.

13. Alzheimer's Society. *One in three people born in 2015 will develop dementia, new analysis shows.* http://www.alzheimersresearchuk.org/one-in-three-2015-develop-dementia/ (accessed 22 June 2017).

14. Mortimer JL. Significant Absences: Faulkner's Rhetoric of Loss. *Novel: A Forum on Fiction* 1981; 14(3): 232-250.

15. Jordan M. *The Essential Guide to Avoiding Dementia.* Hammersmith Books; 2013.

16. Livinston G, Sommerlad A, Orgeta V et al. Dementia prevention, intervention, and care: The Lancet Commissions *The Lancet* 20 July 2017. doi.org/10.1016/S0140-6736(17)31363-6.

17. Sixsmith A, Stilwell J, Copeland J. 'Rementia': Challenging the limits of dementia care. *International Journal of Geriatric Psychiatry* 1993; 8(12): 993-1000.

Chapter 3

Happiness in dementia

Summary

- Technology (at least at its present level) is of limited help to people with dementia.

- People with dementia need above all contact with others and continued interaction with wider society.

- Acceptance by society is vital and current initiatives to promote this are helpful.

- Depression is often accepted by health professionals as inevitable for people with dementia, but evidence does not always show that people with dementia feel depressed – although carers may do so.

- Quality of life in dementia does not depend on memory.

- Despite losses of cognition and function, quality of life and personhood remain resilient for most people with dementia.

- Quality of life is often assessed positively by people with dementia and may even improve as dementia progresses.

- Stories written by people with dementia often yield a positive message not usually conveyed by traditional medical texts.

- Maintaining a sense of citizenship and meaning appears important for wellbeing with or without dementia.

I. (MARY)

In this chapter we air a basic difference of opinion. Noel thinks that most people with dementia (PwD) are happy – I do not. In my experience, most PwD are not happy – but they should be able to be if society were more supportive towards them. To consider this further, it is necessary first to look at what dementia really means. I think it is important to get away from the common, mythical approach of both the media and many medical professionals that dementia is all about memory. It is not. Dementia is about function. Many of us have poor memories and those who do often become adept at using aids to prompt their memory: lists, reminders, calendars and, increasingly, various forms of technology. Indeed, many of us who have no diagnosis of dementia would be hard put to manage without electronic devices, which have become so necessary in the past few years. It can be hard to imagine getting by without our email, our mobile phones and our satnavs, or to recall how we were once able to keep in touch with friends and relatives before Facebook, Instagram and Skype.

There is nothing wrong with using aids to assist a poor memory and needing to use them does not indicate dementia. If I have a bad memory it may be that I cannot immediately recall today's date. But I am able to work it out by checking a calendar or remembering that yesterday was Monday 3rd and so today must be the 4th, or recalling that Friday was my daughter's birthday and counting forward from that.

Ability to function in everyday life

So, a poor memory alone is not actually a prime symptom of dementia, whatever the media would like us to think. When the diagnostic process is taking place, what is being considered is the ability to function in day-to-day life independently (once physical disability is excluded).

- Can the person wash and dress him/herself?

- Can they manage their finances?

- Are they able to use everyday equipment like washing machines, telephones and remote controls?

- Can they prepare a simple meal and make a hot drink?

- Are they able to find their way around in familiar neighbourhoods?

In other words, are they able to function independently in normal, everyday life? The clearest division between memory impairment due to age, mild cognitive impairment (MCI) or illness, and dementia is the ability to function in the everyday world.

Generally, PwD have an understanding that they used to be able to change channels with the remote control, follow a recipe to bake a cake, or understand how to use the shower. They know that they *should* be able to do these things – after all they have done them for many years without thinking. When they discover that they cannot do these things they are often cross, unhappy and bewildered. They cannot work out what is wrong. If asked, most PwD will claim that they still can do all these things – because they recall being able to do them.

There are many aids and appliances, many different types of technological equipment which can help with both memory and function. Many of us are familiar with assisted technology in the shape of call alarms, sensor pads and door alarms. People can now get their drugs dispensed in 'dosette packs' which are labelled to assist with regular medication. Cameras and recording equipment can help to identify those who call at the door. GPS equipment can help to pinpoint the location of someone wearing a personal monitor. Alarms can prompt those who have poor memory to eat, keep appointments and take medication. However, none of this technology works as well to help those with cognitive problems as the presence of help and support in the form of other people.

As mentioned in Chapter 2, the three things which are known to slow the progress of dementia, and to help those with dementia to function well in society, are a reduction in stress, physical exercise and, above all, social contact.

The importance of social contact

In the early stages of dementia – before diagnosis even – those who are affected frequently begin to avoid social contact. Yet it is continuing social contact and interaction with others that is known to help slow cognitive decline more than any other one factor.[1] It is important to encourage those with MCI or early-stage dementia to mix with others and play a part in social events.

The reason social contact is avoided or restricted is usually due to stress. The person with cognitive problems becomes aware of difficulties in following conversations, taking part in debate and discussion, keeping track of what is being said; and the usual response is to draw back from social contact, avoid situations where these difficulties become obvious and restrict oneself to familiar people, places and events. Some people, even in this early stage, stop going out at all, or refuse to attend any social event unless accompanied by a close family member or friend whom they trust and rely on. If society in general is to become more supportive of those with dementia, then this is an area which needs to be addressed. How can we make a society where those with dementia are encouraged to continue to play a part in the community around them?

What is helpful?

To address this question I would suggest that we look at day centre care for PwD. This may seem an odd suggestion as day care probably brings to mind the idea of segregation, of 'hiding away' and setting PwD apart. The reason I suggest starting in this area is because of one major important fact, which is that most PwD who attend a day centre really enjoy their time there.

It is true that many resist the suggestion to begin attending and, indeed, may make difficulties to begin with, but there are two main reasons for that. The first, and most important, is the fact that attending a day centre is a new experience, and involves meeting new people, learning new ways and finding the way in unfamiliar surroundings. All of this is stressful for PwD and the natural reaction is to resist being exposed to stress. But over time the place, people and activities become familiar and the stress is negated.

The second reason for early difficulties may be the reaction of the main carer. Often when I suggest day care, it is the carer who balks. This needs to be addressed separately, and the carer encouraged to see what is in the best interests of the one they care for. Once settled in the day centre, the most interesting factor is that PwD really enjoy their time there, look forward to it (as far as they are able), and get a huge amount of satisfaction from their time there. Why? I have researched this and talked often to PwD who attend day centres. It seems that what matters most is the fact that when attending a day centre PwD feel at ease, they are less stressed than when trying to make their way in general society. Indeed, the comment of one user that 'Everyone understands there – I can be myself' encapsulates how PwD feel. They can relax and just enjoy their time without constantly having to feel that they have to 'keep up' with those around them, or strain to understand the conversations going on, or get bewildered because they don't know what to do or in which direction to go.

We see the same thing in dementia cafés, which used to be run by the Alzheimer's Society around the country. These services are meant for both the carer and for the PwD, and they all run in slightly different ways but, just as with day centres, dementia cafés prove popular with PwD because they are places where they can go and feel accepted and under less stress. Because all are taking part in activities together, PwD still feel part of society – they feel more 'normal'.

Now, this chapter is not about the benefits or otherwise of day centres or dementia cafés for PwD. I have written the above simply to point out that although PwD are frequently confused, over-stressed and unhappy when trying to take part in social life, when attending the day centre or the dementia café they are less confused, less stressed and often happy. Surely our aim should be to create a situation where this can be the case most of the time; to ensure that PwD can live well and continue to enjoy the society of others and the occupations and activities that they prefer. If this can happen sometimes (as at the day centre) could we not aim to ensure that it is possible most of the time?

What do we as a society need to do to assist happiness in dementia?

Some things are already being done. In many places, in Britain at least, there is a huge campaign to make businesses, shops and public areas 'dementia friendly'. The 'Dementia friends' campaign by the Alzheimer's Society has also had a big impact in terms of making people generally aware of the difficulties experienced by those with dementia trying to function in everyday life. These are all good initiatives. But acceptance is the key. The above initiatives make people aware of dementia and they may make people more willing to help when they see someone having difficulties, but do they make PwD more accepted?

People with dementia try to cover up their difficulties

Someone who experiences a pain in their leg is likely to consult a doctor to try to find out what is wrong; they may accept a referral to a specialist consultant and have the problem investigated by X-rays, scans and other methods. When they visit their doctor, they are unlikely to say that they feel no pain and that they can walk without difficulty. Someone who is experiencing cognitive difficulties may voluntarily consult a doctor, but it is more likely that a close relative will make the appointment for them or nag them into attending. At the doctor's it is very likely that they will make light of their problem, will tell the doctor that they have few difficulties, can manage all everyday activities and that (although they may have a little memory problem) all the worries of their relatives are negligible and the result only of 'getting old'. Partly this is because PwD have difficulty in recognising their own cognitive problems, but partly this 'denial' and attempt to 'cover up' is due to the fact that to have cognitive problems is to be stigmatised. Society still sees PwD as mad, un-balanced and foolish.

People with dementia don't ask for help and may even reject it when offered

People with dementia seldom ask for help and may often reject it when offered. This is partly because they only remember what they used to be able to do, and they genuinely feel they do not need extra attention. But it is also partly because to admit the need for help with quite ordinary everyday things again suggests foolishness and vulnerability.

Many people have a basic misunderstanding of the condition of dementia and their attempts to help are based on this. They think that because they (in their condition without symptoms of dementia) can understand that help is needed by those with cognitive difficulties, then so will those who have the condition understand that they need help. But as a general rule, you cannot explain to PwD how they can help themselves. Even medical and social care professionals frequently don't understand this basic fact. I have had a social care professional asking for my help say: 'How do I explain to Mrs X that if we de-clutter her bathroom she will be more likely to use it?' The fact is, it is not the clutter that is preventing Mrs X from having a wash.

I have heard a politician say that now he 'understands dementia' then if he is afflicted he will be happy to accept help. I am very sure that if those circumstances arise he will not. I have even heard a consultant psychiatrist specialising in dementia tell me that: 'She says she is managing her finances so I don't think there is a problem.' A week later this lady was picked up by the police for driving without insurance.

People with dementia need acceptance like everyone else

People with dementia frequently don't feel any different from how they were before diagnosis, and they do not want to be made to feel different. Yes, they need (rather than want) help and support, but they want above all to still feel part of society, to have a function and a place. In day centres and dementia cafés, PwD are accepted and made to feel comfortable, and this is good and helpful, but these services still set PwD apart. Those who have a diagnosis are still a part of society and they continue to want to feel a part of society – to feel 'normal'.

Everyone can help here. Is it so difficult to allow someone with cognitive problems to continue to be part of your social group, to listen to them with the same courtesy that you give to those without obvious symptoms, to continue to accept their company and to give some unobtrusive help if required? My challenge would be to all the social and community groups – to the WI, to the Rotary clubs, to U3A, to church groups and social and political clubs, to community choirs and keep-fit groups – to all these local community networks. Accept PwD and give them a place within your group, just as you would accept those with an obvious physical disability. Help and support those with cognitive problems. Allow them to continue to feel part of society as a whole. One day it may be you who needs this acceptance.

II. (NOEL)

Mood and dementia

There has been considerable research looking at mood and depression in dementia. Depression is often assumed to be an inevitable consequence of the condition. Medical texts on dementia emphasise that PwD are more likely to suffer depression than those without. For example, it has been observed that around 30 per cent of patients with Alzheimer's disease display depressive symptoms and 20 per cent are clinically depressed.[1] Depression is therefore often viewed as a neuropsychiatric complication, or 'non-cognitive feature' of dementia, one that is directly linked to the pathology of specific areas in the brain. For example, one research paper saw an 'observed disproportionate loss of noradrenergic and cholinergic neurons in the LC and basal nucleus of Meynert [that] may represent an important organic substrate of depression in AD'.[2] Depression in vascular dementia is also thought to be directly linked to vascular changes in the brain.[3] However, suggesting that low mood in dementia is a direct neuropsychiatric consequence of dementia-related pathological changes in the brain is too simplistic, and does not provide any insight into how people experience and navigate the challenges associated with the condition.

Quality of life in dementia is not simple

'Quality of life' (QoL) is an important concept when looking at the effect of dementia on people's lives. QoL reflects a person's subjective sense of wellbeing, rather than symptom scales or memory scores, which do not reflect how a person actually feels about their life. QoL is a nebulous concept, which varies from person to person and culture to culture, but includes a number of components such as physical and psychological health, level of independence, social relationships, the environment and personal beliefs.[4] Although difficult to define, it is important to consider, as healthcare's main aim is to improve QoL and wellbeing and not memory score. But what do we know of QoL in dementia? Is it solely dependent on mood? Does it decline in a predictable and linear fashion with memory? Whilst mood affects QoL,[5] it is not the whole picture, as we shall see later.

QoL in dementia has traditionally been measured according to carer perception

Until relatively recently, the QoL of a PwD has been measured from others' points of view, generally a carer or outside observer. The rationale for this approach was that traditionally dementia tended to be diagnosed later, and it was assumed that people with more advanced dementia were unable to articulate how they felt about their lives, or that their perceptions were somehow not valid. If PwD were to display humour about their condition, or talk about their past or their present, they were assumed to be in denial regarding their condition or their lives.[6] But, QoL is now accepted to be a highly personal and subjective concept, and external 'objective' observations do not reflect the real picture.[7] For example, in a study by Hoe et al, when perceptions of QoL from the perspective of both carers and PwD were examined, there were some interesting differences. Whilst a PwD's view of their QoL was strongly linked to their mood, most carers believed that QoL was most related to dependency and disability. This discrepancy succinctly illustrated that carers tended to project their own assumptions regarding QoL, rather than considering the concept from the perspective of the person they were caring for.[8]

Similarly, focus groups have shown that PwD had higher hopes for their QoL than their caregivers did for them.[7] This hope expressed by PwD is not mis-founded, as Hoe et al's study showed that whilst QoL was strongly influenced by mood, it did not necessarily diminish as dementia progressed.[9] This raises the question of what effect a care giver's more negative predictions of QoL can have on the person they are caring for, and in particular, whether it becomes self-actualising.

What do people with dementia actually say about their lives?

What has been curiously absent in the scientific debate about QoL in dementia, until fairly recently, has been the perspective of people actually living with dementia. When you start to look at the issue of QoL in dementia from the perspective of people affected themselves, rich evidence emerges. And in particular, the assumption of 'depression' and a pervasively negative experience in dementia is challenged. As stated previously, a person's subjective rating of their own state is the gold standard for measuring QoL.[8] When PwD are actually asked about their situation and the quality of their lives, the story is more positive than we have been led to believe from other people's accounts. For example, Steeman et al looked into the question and listened to the perspectives of 20 older people living with dementia.[6]

They uncovered numerous positive accounts of resilience, humour and fortitude, rather than expected narratives of inevitable decay and despair. They remark that in their study 'living with dementia was often presented as a positive narrative, one that told of only minor problems and which stressed abilities and contentment with life. Being valued, rather than losing one's cognition or identity was central in their experience … More in-depth analyses of participants' narratives revealed, however, that they were constantly balancing their feelings of value and worthlessness, struggling to remain someone of value. This struggle was prompted by threats posed by dementia and by the persons' interactions with others.[6] Their later point echoes Mary's sentiment that maintaining social connections in dementia is of vital importance in maintaining QoL. Steeman et al. also commented that whilst these positive stories of PwD can be superficially interpreted as denial or lack of awareness due to cognitive impairment, the narratives revealed active attempts to 'counterbalance devaluation'.[6]

Other recent research documenting the stories of PwD supports the findings by Steeman et al that when PwD provide positive accounts of their lives, they are not simply in denial. A study by Werezak and Stewart found that PwD displayed a striking openness, and wanted to be educated about the illness to successfully assimilate it into their lives.[10] Many also reported that a perceived lack of support from friends and family hindered their success in accepting the condition. Another study by Moyle et al emphasises the importance of the quality of family and other relationships in the QoL of PwD.[11] In their study of PwD who had moved into nursing and residential care, they found that the main factors that maintained a positive QoL included feeling in control of life, being able to contribute to their new community, and maintaining positive relationships with family. When people felt of little use and value to society, their QoL suffered. Moyle suggested that it was important 'to understand how relationships might be maintained and strengthened following a move into long-term care and ... the importance of control and its influence on feeling valued'.[11] What is notably absent from these accounts of active attempts to maintaining identity, self-worth and meaning in life, are references to memory and daily function. Whilst they are part of the story, they are not the most important part, when stories from PwD are actually considered.

What happens as dementia progresses?

Whilst traditional discourses on dementia generally position PwD as a victim, with inevitable pain and personality disintegration at the end, this is not borne out by research looking at QoL. Whilst increasing severity of dementia is associated with changes in ability to express a positive 'effect' or mood, it is observed that when people enter more severe stages, there is an upswing of contentment and pleasure and less worry.[12] QoL is also observed to increase when the level of dementia is more severe.[13] This has been assumed to be due to neuronal loss and structural changes in the brain leading to impaired insight into the predicament of one's position, but there is no evidence to support this idea. And despite increasing dependency, people with severe dementia are generally content.[12,13]

I routinely explain this in my memory clinic, saying that even as dementia worsens, most people are pretty happy if they are in receipt of appropriate care. Despite this, carers may project their own values regarding dependence on the loved PwD, with a prevalent assumption that they could never be happy or enjoy life if they were that dependent on care from others. I think this assumption is rooted in Western culture, whereas other cultures accept interdependency as an important aspect of life.[4]

The prevalent message that emerges from accounts of PwD is that overall QoL remains robust, or can even increase, in dementia. Despite reductions in independence and cognitive ability, PwD generally remained 'optimistic about their quality of life, valued being able to reminisce about the past and also managed to make the best of it and take one day at the time'.[5] However, pre-morbid personality traits and general outlook influence a person's ability to remain positive and enjoy life in the face of dementia.[5] Selwood et al explain that 'mood and personality factors have a strong influence on the way we perceive our life and that despite changes in circumstances which will inevitably occur ... people will assimilate these changes into their view of their life and the world.'[5]

Welcome to our world

I think that the best evidence of the resilience of the human spirit in dementia comes from the experiences of PwD themselves. A recent anthology of 'life writing' by PwD is entitled *Welcome to Our World*.[14] What is surprising is that this recent book is the first collection of stories to give a voice to PwD. In it, eight individuals in a life-writing exercise group, supported by trainee psychologists, tell their individual stories. It is an excellent book and probably one of the most helpful texts that anyone newly diagnosed can read. As Keith Oliver, who writes the preface and one of the chapters (and the Foreword to our book), explains, 'what makes this book unique is that it is written by a group of people who each have a diagnosis of dementia, who want to share some stories from their lives alongside expressing some thoughts surrounding inhabiting the world of dementia from inside.'[14] Like Jo Brand, who wrote the Foreword, I also found the narratives contained within the book to be 'so pragmatic, joyful and positive that it is hard not to be swept along by their enthusiasm'.[14]

The stories, although they include feelings of shock and sorrow at being diagnosed with dementia, also describe tales of reliance, optimism and contentment in the face of the diagnosis. Reading these accounts powerfully neutralises the idea that PwD have little meaning or quality in their lives. In a preface written by the psychology students who assisted the writers in compiling their stories, they remark that although 'the medical definition of dementia tells us that it is degenerative; that cognitive and social function diminished over time. This seems in direct contradiction to our own experiences. We have gained a greater understanding of the tragedies, comedies, loves and losses that make up the tapestry of human experience.'[14] Reading the accounts of living with dementia in *Welcome to Our World* provides not only a sense of optimism in dementia, but also pragmatic advice to maintain quality and meaning in life. In the book, B de Frene vividly details a number of periods in her life, and also goes on to show how meaning can reside not only in preserved fragments of memory, but also in more random thoughts and feelings. Her poetic musings demonstrate a mind still active and a life still lived.

Similarly, Chris R's writing shows an identity that has subsumed dementia, and not the other way round. The title of his chapter, 'Me and my dementia', illustrates the direction of ownership and a determinism that although he 'may have dementia ...dementia does not have [him]!'.[14] The book not only demonstrates the preserved spirit of the authors, but also a wisdom in how to live with dementia. Another contributor, Charles, provides a clear battle plan, including a testimonial on the value of meditation and a remarkable account of the value of music. I would imagine that if Charles ever experienced agitation at a later stage of his dementia, his chapter provides a clear personalised prescription of what pieces of music might be played to calm him by his carers rather than resorting to medication. Lastly, Chris N reminds us of the important adage that life is not a destination, but a journey and how dementia has prompted him 'to view ... life in a very different way and learn to live for, and in, the moment'.[14] The writers acknowledge the help of the psychology students in bringing out the best in them 'with gentleness and understanding'. I only wish that this support to find meaning in the dementia experience was routinely available to all living with the condition.

Conclusions

Mary makes a number of points that I agree with – that dementia is not only about memory, and that maintaining social connections is of prime importance. We disagree whether most PwD are happy. But I think it is important to emphasise to PwD, especially at the time of diagnosis, that existing qualitative research examining QoL in dementia and narratives from PwD themselves yield a surprisingly positive message which is not usually conveyed in traditional medical texts and discourse – namely, that despite expected declines in both cognition and function, QoL and personhood remain resilient in dementia. It may be that mine and Mary's differing views are explained by the different groups of people that we see at different stage of their dementia journey.

Mary most often sees people adjusting to a relatively new diagnosis of dementia, whilst I tend to see people in more advanced stages of the disease, where adjustment has occurred. It could be that once people accept their dementia, and have successfully navigated all the practical social care hurdles of brokering care to mobilise appropriate support, they are then able to finally get on with living and being themselves. The reverse also holds in that when PwD are unsupported and left alone, they lose a sense of themselves and are unhappy. This goes back to one of Mary's initial points that I wholeheartedly support: that most PwD have the potential to be happy if the rest of us help them to achieve this.

REFERENCES

1. Allen N, Burns A. The noncognitive features of dementia. *Reviews in clinical gerontology* 1995; 5(01): 57-75.

2. Förstl H, Burns A, Luthert P, et al. Clinical and neuropathological correlates of depression in Alzheimer's disease. *Psychological Medicine* 1992; 22(04): 877-84.

3. Ballard C, McKeith I, O'Brien J, et al. Neuropathological substrates of dementia and depression in vascular dementia, with a particular focus on cases with small infarct volumes. *Dementia and Geriatric Cognitive Disorders* 2000; 11(2): 59-65.

4. WHO. The World Health Organization quality of life assessment (WHOQOL): position paper from the World Health Organization. *Social Science & Medicine* 1995; 41(10): 1403-09.

5. Selwood A, Thorgrimsen L, Orrell M. Quality of life in dementia – a one-year follow-up study. *International Journal of Geriatric Psychiatry* 2005; 20(3): 232-37.

6. Steeman E, Godderis J, Grypdonck M, et al. Living with dementia

from the perspective of older people: is it a positive story? *Aging Mental Health* 2007; 11(2): 119-30.

7.   Thorgrimsen L, Selwood A, Spector A, et al. Whose quality of life is it anyway?: The validity and reliability of the Quality of Life-Alzheimer's Disease (QoL-AD) scale. *Alzheimer Disease & Associated Disorders* 2003; 17(4): 201-08.

8.   Hoe J, Hancock G, Livingston G, et al. Quality of life of people with dementia in residential care homes. *The British Journal of Psychiatry* 2006; 188(5): 460-64.

9.   Hoe J, Hancock G, Livingston G, et al. Changes in the quality of life of people with dementia living in care homes. *Alzheimer Disease and Associated Disorders* 2009; 23(3): 285.

10. Werezak L, Stewart N. Learning to live with early dementia. *The Canadian Journal of Nursing Research* 2002; 34(1): 67-85.

11. Moyle W, Venturto L, Griffiths S, et al. Factors influencing quality of life for people with dementia: A qualitative perspective. *Aging & Mental Health* 2011; 15(8): 970-77.

12. Albert SM, Jacobs DM, Sano M, et al. Longitudinal study of quality of life in people with advanced Alzheimer's disease. *The American Journal of Geriatric Psychiatry* 2001; 9(2): 160-68.

13. Zank S, Leipold B. The relationship between severity of dementia and subjective well-being. *Aging & Mental Health* 2001; 5(2): 191-96.

14. Nots FM. *Welcome to Our World: A Collection of Life Writing by People Living with Dementia*. London: Alzheimer's Society; 2014.

Chapter 4

Maintaining ourselves in dementia

Summary

- Medicine rarely considers the effect of dementia on the individual's sense of themselves.

- Sociological models of the self challenge the widespread notion that the loss of memory in dementia equates with a loss of the self.

- Understanding that 'the self' has many parts is key in understanding its resilience in the face of dementia.

- Our memories serve our sense of self, not the other way around.

- Whilst the intellectual and narrative self may be impaired by dementia, the social self and embodied self are resilient.

- The threat to the self in dementia occurs when the diagnosis becomes a preoccupying label that affects the quality of social interactions with others.

- Kitwood describes a stage early in the course of dementia where a person can improve or decline, depending on how the social network of the person responds.

- Our self-concept naturally changes during the course of our lives. Cultivating a flexible sense of self-identity is an important defence against dementia.

- An excessive focus on risk mitigation can dampen the self, just as some self-affirming activities can be risky. A balance needs to be struck.

- Maintaining social interactions, being open to multiple facets of the self, being mindful of threats to the self and prioritising the self above other considerations, such as risk, may all help preserve the individual in the face of dementia.

I. (NOEL)

What constitutes our sense of self? What are the core parts of our being? Are we defined by our memories? If we lose our memory, do we lose our sense of self? These existential questions are at the heart of the fear of dementia but are rarely examined by medicine and the medical model of dementia. Although there is increasing interest in these important questions in the sociological literature, most clinicians and carers working with people with dementia (PwD) are generally unaware that this discourse exists. This means that this critical debate regarding the self and dementia is rarely ever shared with PwD and their families. This is a missed opportunity to confront a primal fear of dementia head on, and also to share an alternative and more optimistic perspective of dementia. My experience of sharing these concepts with PwD, alongside medical information, is positive – not just in terms of giving details of some heartening research, which argues that the self is preserved in dementia, but also in explicitly demonstrating that the social and psychological aspects of dementia are as important as the biological.

The aim of this chapter is to introduce the social theory relating to the self and dementia and to challenge the widespread notion that loss of memory in dementia equates with a loss of self. The research in this area provides new insights into how PwD maintain a sense of identity in creative and dynamic ways. This is in contrast with the populist nihilistic ideas that as memory declines, self-hood also diminishes in an inevitable linear fashion. Common threats to the self in dementia will also be discussed as well as potential ways to manage these threats. By the end of this chapter it is hoped that your concept of the self may have broadened to a more encompassing definition, one that is more resilient to the challenges posed by dementia. For the purposes of coherence, the terms 'self', 'identity' and 'self-hood' are used interchangeably to imply the individual person.

Our multiple selves

Before the effect of dementia on the self can be considered, we need to define 'the self'. The Merriam-Webster dictionary defines it in terms of reflexive personal pronouns – myself, himself, herself.[1] An online search using the question 'what is the self?' brings up more expansive psychological, philosophical and spiritual definitions. For example, one definition equates the self with identity, as:

> That being which is the source of consciousness, the agent responsible for an individual's thoughts and actions, or the substantial nature of a person which endures and unifies consciousness over time.[2]

Even this definition feels somewhat unsatisfactory. It is clear that the concept of the self has a number of components, such as consciousness, agency (control), attributes, individuality, values, roles and relationships.

Understanding the range of concepts which constitute the self is key in understanding its resilience in the face of the dementia. It is also clear that even though the self is difficult to define, most people have an intuitive sense of themselves and what defines them as an individual. The onset of an illness like dementia forces us to define ourselves in clearer terms. It makes us urgently consider who we are and what makes us who we are. If we define ourselves in narrow terms based on intellect or autonomy throughout our lives, there may be significant anticipatory grief regarding the loss of the self soon after the onset of dementia. This sudden confrontation with existential issues in dementia is made more acute by the general avoidance of discourse on life and death, and the value system in Western society being focused on the importance of self-determinism and individualism. Fear regarding future incapacity or dependence on others brought about by dementia thereby becomes an automatic socially conditioned fear.

Our social selves

Whilst independence and autonomy are highly prized human attributes in Western culture, do these qualities actually define who we are? Our inherent social nature and interdependence with family and friends are manifest across the whole human lifespan. We live in a rich social network and in relation to others. We do not usually reside in a social vacuum. We define ourselves in the context of relationships to others. We are not just an individual, but also a wife, a son, a husband, a sister, a teacher or a friend. Our societal roles and social selves change naturally over the lifespan due to life events, such as divorce, bereavement or illness like dementia. Although our sense of self-identity can be threatened by these multiple life events, our innate nature as social beings remain resilient.

Even if in the final stages of dementia autobiographical memory is completely lost, and a child is not recognised when visiting his/her mother with dementia in a nursing home, this does not automatically invalidate her status as parent. Meaningful and compassionate social interactions between two people are not dependent on cognition and a mutual orientation to role. We instinctively interact with young children, who are naive to their social context, in a positive and unconditional manner; we can adopt the same approach to PwD and remember that positive social interactions have inherent value, irrespective of the cognitive status of the person and perceptions of identity.

It is helpful to know that whilst dementia can erode autobiographical memory, it does not erode our inherently social nature. We remain social creatures and part of social networks to our last breath. I think that everyone should be encouraged to explore concepts of the social self and self-worth, prior to when onset of an illness like dementia forces them to do so. At that point, there may be decreased cognitive reserve, which may make it more difficult to reflect on the flexible nature and value of the social self.

How is the self related to memory?

Are we the sum of our memories? If our memories could be installed into a clone of ourselves, would that other copy be an identical version? Conversely, if we lose our memories, do we stop being ourselves? These questions are posed more often in science fiction than in science or medicine. But, if these questions were addressed in dementia care, then a major fear associated with dementia could be tackled head on. Whilst most people would agree that memories are an important part of who we are, the ways that the self and memory interact are complicated.

I found a number of papers helpful whilst researching the self

The research

Rapaport in 1942 theorised that the self is not an end summation of objective and factually correct autobiographical memories. Rather, he believed that specific memories are stored and filed, according to the needs of the individual to maintain a sense of self.[3]

Another later researcher, Conway, described this complex and active relationship between 'self and memory' in a 2005 paper, where he proposed a 'dynamic self memory system'.[4] In it, he described the variety of methods used to keep our memories coherent with our concept of self. Whilst memories are thought to be the 'database' of the self, it is memory that serves the self, rather than the self being a slave of memory.

in dementia and these are summarised in text boxes as I work through the concepts in the sections that follow.

The concept that the self exists separately from memory has considerable relevance to dementia, where an assumption exists that self simply degrades in a simple linear fashion with declining memory. There have been some recent representations of dementia, such as that in the book and movie, *Still Alice*,[21] which presents an opposing perspective, showing how the self, even stripped of memory and language, remains stoically fluent in the most important of human emotions – love. However, medicine remains generally silent on the issue.

The self in dementia care

Although health and social care attempt to be 'person centred', often the most fundamental processes within health and social care systems undermine the self. From first contact, the concept of self can be side-lined, as from the point of diagnosis the medical narrative is focused on deficit and decline. A person referred to a memory clinic is initially defined by what cannot be done, rather than what can – by what faculties are lost, rather than what is maintained. The concept of self thereby becomes conflated with other more measurable quantities, such as cognitive scores. There will naturally be assumptions made by staff about a patient with a recorded 'normal' mini-mental state examination (MMSE)* of 29, for example, as opposed to someone who has a low score of 3. Medical assessment by its very nature divides individuals into groups and categories. Dementia versus normal. Dementia versus mild cognitive impairment. Labels based on diagnosis, cognitive performance, agency and function are applied, and acted on.

Although this labelling has medical utility and is well intended, it has unintended consequences on self-hood. As Mary and I agreed in Chapter 2, a diagnosis of dementia is not always helpful. Although it can help make sense of difficulties and be used as a starting point for help, the application of the diagnosis can assume a 'master status' which eclipses the individual. Research shows that status assessments of the individual as being mentally incapable, at risk at home, or dependent, all divert attention away from the person.

We have looked at how the self defies simple definition. We know that there is more to the self than just memory and the self may be resilient despite the cognitive impairment that occurs in dementia. Although biomedicine has largely ignored the question of what happens to the self in dementia, the question is increasingly posed by social science. I had worked in the field

*Footnote: The MMSE is the cognitive test that is probably most widely used as a screening tool for dementia.

The research

Touhy suggests that the 'master status' of an Alzheimer's diagnosis may worsen subsequent care through the loss of personhood.[5]

Doyle et al note the process of 'othering',[6] which Touhy says leads to carers only seeing dementia rather than the person.[5]

Other researchers, Beard et al, caution that the 'medicalisation of memory and memory loss may lead to individual narratives being forgotten'.[7]

of dementia, as a memory specialist, for six years and had rarely considered the question myself. I found myself asking this more openly in my conversations with Mary and my patients in the memory clinic. Before this, I realised my silence on the issue in consultations could be interpreted as my being complicit with the automatic assumption of inevitable decline and destruction of the self from dementia. I had noticed this unspoken fear, often present in the consulting room on the faces of relatives and carers, at the point of diagnosis.

But what is actually known about self-preservation in dementia, and where as a doctor could I find out? Although I was aware of the principles of person-centred care, I had never participated in any conversation with medical colleagues about whether dementia threatens the self. Instead, most conversations with other doctors were dominated by discussion of new brain imaging techniques to improve diagnosis, medication to control behavioural aspects of the disease and the promises of new disease-modifying agents always just around the corner. It was only when I was researching this book that I uncovered the debate on the issue.

I would like now to discuss some theories regarding the self in dementia, which these days I try to introduce to patients at the point of diagnosis. People pause to consider this narrative, in a curious and reflective way, similarly to when I first interacted with the material. This dialogue is not an alternative to more traditional medical discourse with patients about further options and support, but it forms an important adjunct even at early stages of the diagnostic process. My sense is that it can powerfully neutralise the 'rhetoric of loss' and therapeutic nihilism that can exist in both patient and practitioner.

The social self in dementia

The research emphasises that relationships are important to us, and this continues even when we are diagnosed with dementia. We define ourselves in relation to others. What people think of us is important. And how we treat others, and how they treat us, can define who we are. We all have direct experiences of how positive social interactions can enrich our lives and how negative experiences of being ignored or undermined can diminish them. This does not change after a dementia diagnosis. Positive social interactions may be even more important during dementia.

As I write this, I reflect on my own life. Some of my social identities, such as being a practising doctor, being a friend of 'x', a member of a swimming club, will at some point end, due to life circumstances such as retirement, relocation and/or frailty. Others may also be threatened by the onset of dementia. However, even if I develop Alzheimer's disease in 30 or 40 years' time, I will always be a (retired) doctor, a husband, a son, and a brother and friend. These social selves will endure, even if my memory and my spoken language are impaired.

I also hope that, if I become a resident of a nursing home, some new social identities will form in my new environment. I hope that even if I lose some of my memories and words, other social aspects of my personality will prosper in my daily interactions with other residents and carers. I hope that I will be regarded as a person who is kind and enjoys rabbiting on about science fiction, even if I am easily frustrated by loud morning television and weak tea. What I also hope is that it will become quickly clear to others around me how much I value my relationships, both old and new. And that even if I have difficulties remembering recent conversations and past events, it is clear to everyone around me

The research

A 2010 review by Caddell and Clare[8] provides an overview of a number of theories regarding the conceptualisation of the self in dementia. One of these is the 'social constructionist' perspective, which describes how the self is constructed and maintained socially. This goes back to a very basic idea that humans are social, not solitary, creatures.

Another researcher, Marks, reminded us in 1997 that 'all human societies are characterised by interdependence. No person is completely self-reliant, since we all (unless we are Robinson Crusoe) live in communities.'[9]

The social constructionist theory of self, developed by Sabat and Harré in 1992,[10] emphasises this and how loss of the social self in dementia occurs as a result of isolation rather than as a direct consequence of brain pathology or amyloid plaques. Sabat and others argue that during our lives we maintain a 'repertoire' of selves through social interactions and relationships. The process of forming multiple social selves and relationships, as fundamental as breathing, does not stop after the onset of dementia. These multiple social selves or role identities do not rely on memory.

This important interplay between biology and the

social world was originally proposed by Kitwood in 1990[11] and will be examined in more detail later in the chapter.

Another model of the self that argues for the maintenance of identity in dementia, is that of the 'embodied self' proposed by Kontos.[12]

She argues that the self does not just reside in the brain's cognitive and contemplative processes, but rather because it is such a fundamental aspect of ourselves, it is also located in the body. Our personhood is not dependent on verbal communication. Even if pre-morbid 'higher level' cognitive and executive abilities are lost, the body continues naturally to express the self.

Kontos's theory of the embodied self in dementia was developed through extensive and detailed observation of the spontaneous interactions between nursing home residents with varying stages of dementia for over eight months. Even for people with very advanced dementia, their ability to interact meaningfully with others was preserved, even in the absence of spoken language.

Kontos believes that our concept of self – the embodied self – is resilient to dementia even in the final stages. Even if the mind cannot fully express the self, the body knows what to do. This simple yet profound idea neutralises the catastrophic fear of dementia as a dehumanising agent. I first read her papers several years ago, and am a great believer in her work. I think her ideas offer as much hope and optimism for those affected by dementia as any biomedical research that I have read in recent years regarding medications and potential disease-modifying agents. I also agree with Kontos that many carers intuitively know this, and her theories may help this group validate their interactions and caring experiences.

that my interactions with them are important to me as a social person.

To recap, there is a divide between how the biomedical and sociological models consider the self in dementia. Medicine rarely considers the effect of dementia on the individual self. Instead, medical discourses are dominated by diagnosis, assessment of risk, function and capacity and 'evidence-based' treatment. These concerns tend to eclipse consideration of the individual, and as a result, the self can be conflated with memory and assumed to decline in parallel. But, the link between the progress of cognitive impairment and the deterioration of self is not proven.[8]

Most sociological models of self in dementia support the idea of preservation of the self. These models provide a more positive perspective than the pure biomedical model, which is often focused on risk, deficit and decline. These models also emphasise that there are many components of the self and whilst dementia can alter these, they are not completely lost. Whilst the intellectual and narrative self may be impaired, the social self and the embodied self are resilient to dementia, even in later stages.

Even when cognition and memory are severely impaired, we never lose our intuitive ability to express ourselves through our physical appearance, our responses to others, our instinct to care and to comfort someone in distress, and in our reactions to dance and music.[12] The latter example is famously demonstrated in a documentary called *Alive Inside,* featuring a filmed interaction between Henry (a nursing home resident with advanced dementia) and the late neurologist Oliver Sacks. Henry is reawakened when he is played music important in his youth – jazz by singer Cab Calloway.[22] This response has also been referred to as a 'musical embodiment' of the self, another potent example that the self does not purely reside in episodic memory.[13]

These are important positive messages for PwD to hear at all stages of the disease.

Interpretative, social constructionist and biomedical accounts of dementia need not be seen as mutually exclusive. They can be combined meaningfully to improve understanding of the disease and to enhance care and research. Effective clinicians need to be proficient in both the reductionist processes of diagnosis and the more humanistic interpersonal skills needed to relate successfully to PwD. One researcher, Perry, suggests that care can be further improved by repositioning the medical diagnosis *behind* the narrative of the individual patient.[14] We will look at these ideas more closely in the next section.

Kitwood and the maintenance of the social self in dementia

Probably more than any other author, Tom Kitwood has been successful in steering the narrative of dementia away from the

The research

Kitwood argues that there are many potential threats to the individual and self-identity in dementia. Whilst it is often assumed that these are solely biologically driven as the brain's structure is altered by dementia-related brain cell loss and pathology, such as plaques and tangles, many threats to self-identity are in fact social. Kitwood describes the origin of these threats in detail in his seminal paper 'The dialectics of dementia: with particular reference to Alzheimer's disease'.[11] He shows how a dementia diagnosis can become a damaging and preoccupying label that negatively affects a person's interactions with others. He explains that the biology of the brain has effects on how the mind works and is expressed, and that positive interactions with others can also affect the biology of the brain.

disease process and back to the individual.

Kitwood's ideas are similar to the principles behind psychotherapy, where meaningful communication with an empathic other can bring about positive changes in both the recipient's mindset and brain structure. This is still true in dementia. Although brain pathology is significant in dementia, the social self, as well as the life experiences of the person, are equally important. If a person with dementia is marginalised or isolated as dementia progresses, this will have as much, or perhaps more, impact than the pathological changes in the brain. The corollary of this is that people's identity in dementia can be maintained by positive interaction with others.

This has several implications. It implies that the social realm is as important as the biological in dementia. And whilst the biological plaques and tangles may not be amenable to medical intervention, the social realm is always open to change. Kitwood's ideas provide clarity and direction in dementia care. If we treat everyone around us an individual, with inherent self-worth, irrespective of the presence of dementia or not, we can contribute to the maintenance of that person's self-identity.

Kitwood describes a 'meta-stable' state in dementia, where early in the course of the disease, there is a point where a PwD can improve ('rementia') or decline, depending on how the social network around the person responds.[15] If concerted attempts are made to engage the individual with dementia and bolster his/ her sense of individuality and identity, then this will stabilise the condition. Conversely, there are social processes that will accelerate the condition. He says these processes contribute to a 'malignant social psychology'.

Many of these processes come as no surprise, as we have all directly experienced the effect of these at one time or other and know how isolating they can be. Examples include disempowerment, infantilisation, labelling and invalidation. The most dramatic example of these processes occurs in examples of institutional abuse, where residents are bullied and reduced by the simultaneous application of these effects. But these processes can be seen in operation in the mildest of forms, where they can have a significant effect on reducing the individual's sense of identity and autonomy. This often begins at the earliest point of diagnosis, where a relative anxiously wants to shield a loved one from a dementia diagnosis, and wants to talk to the doctor alone when providing a history of cognitive impairment. Although well intended, this earliest example of marginalisation has negative consequences for the individual, and suggests that they are not able to cope with the truth, or that their understanding of their difficulties is not to be trusted and that their status as an autonomous individual is to be questioned.

Later in the illness, in care-home settings, this can progress to infantalisation, where attempts to maintain skills in dressing are disregarded as an impatient carer does up buttons when it is taking too long to do so. However, Kitwood acknowledges that the art of truly nuanced and patient-centred care is dialectical, in that one needs to simultaneously attend to a person's care needs, whilst maintaining and preserving autonomy. This dialectical care is not easy to master, but it can be supported through approaches to care, such as 'dementia care mapping' which he pioneered.

Malignant social psychology in 2017

Kitwood used the phrase 'malignant social psychology' to describe the impact that social processes could have on PwD in the 1990s. What has changed since his seminal work? There is no doubt that his ideas were a watershed in considering the individual in dementia, and many writers have taken his ideas forward. However, the threats to personhood he identified have, in some ways, worsened. Austerity and the state of the world economy, combined with the privatisation and commodification of care, is a big threat to person-centred care. Getting to know individuals and providing person-centred care takes time, and time costs money. Carers in nursing homes are some of the most poorly paid and poorly trained staff in Europe. Nursing homes in the UK are now largely run as money-making businesses and organisational cost pressure translates to less individual time with individual residents. This means that most care interactions focus on basic or personal care, rather than on social interactions, which are vital for maintaining self-identity.

Other factors that exist in the current health care system that I feel could now be added to Kitwood's list of malignant social psychology processes include that of pseudo-inclusion, commodification of dementia and risk myopia. The NHS has become dominated by a management culture that is increasingly focused on the standardisation of process and outcome. Most executive boards within the NHS do not include clinicians, practising or otherwise. Finance, corporate risk, external audit, commissioning, efficiency saving and transformation are the most common words heard at board level. And the notion of the individual patient is rarely considered unless a serious untoward incident or complaint is being addressed. Whilst clinicians on the front-line deal with individuals and individual need, the governance of NHS providers does not always support this care and the individual becomes lost in the complex system of health and social care.

Clinicians' time with individuals is now often encroached on by the need to complete clinical coding, risk assessment tools, care plan protocols and physical screening tools, all of which can be potent distractors from the needs of the person. Many trusts have also corrupted the notion of person-centred care through a process of pseudo-inclusion. Patients can be asked to fill out or sign lengthy statements of care, supposedly to support their individual care needs, yet care is delivered in a standardised tick-box way. Similarly, the increasing neo-liberalisation of the health and social care economy means that care encounters are limited by time and cost. Health and social care providers are often squeezed into providing care at the lowest unit cost. Dementia does not benefit from this commodification of disease. Dementia care can be complicated, time-consuming and relies often on one-to-one support and human interaction rather than a standardised procedure. Dementia care is also relationship-based and involves careful liaison with families and multiple agencies. Good relationships take time to build.

The best ways to preserve the self in dementia

A number of studies have looked at ways to support the self and self-identity in dementia. Most of these studies did not specifically aim to do this, but reported this as a potential positive effect of therapeutic work with PwD, particularly those in nursing homes. These included groups with a focus on art, music or other creative activities. However, some studies have looked more specifically at ways to support individual identity in dementia. These had a number of different approaches – a focus on maintaining existing social roles and exploring new ones, psychotherapy (with an emphasis on self-knowledge, activity and communication) and creation of self-narrative and autobiography through 'life-book' work.[16]

Although these studies initially appear to identify differing strategies, they share some commonalities – namely, an active attempt to engage with the PwD and time with real human contact. These different approaches also build on theories of the self in dementia – namely that we have multiple selves, both in health and in illness: our social selves, our roles and identities, and our past life history and relationships. Any successful strategy to maintain identity in dementia should aim to work on all of these fronts. I will now consider this in more detail.

Be open to new selves

I have spent some time attempting to clarify the notion of the self and identity in dementia. This is an important first step. If we hold a very narrow and restricted definition of self-identity, equated, for example, to our previous occupational role, then this is a high-risk strategy when faced with the onset of dementia. Memory, language and other executive functions that underpin this role identity may indeed be affected by dementia, and if the individual concept of self exists only within this template, then he or she is likely to experience a significant loss of identity with the onset of cognitive impairment.

We naturally flirt with a number of self-identities and roles over the lifespan that define our self-worth. Some of these are linked to past educational, professional and material achievements, whilst others are more rooted in our relationships to others. If we can explore and nourish a range of self-identities that are not all dependent on cognition and achievement, then the onset of dementia should not be as threatening to our sense of self-worth. An example might be that of a retired barrister, who as well as being defined by the achievements and competencies related to an illustrious career, has also embraced other roles to define his or her life in retirement.

Examples could include the barrister developing an identity as a kind and compassionate person to others, as a lover of Beethoven, or a person who likes to look sharp and colourful, or as a kind grandparent. Whilst the identity of a keen legal mind might be threatened by dementia, these other self-identities might remain robust, even in the presence of severe cognitive impairment. Hence, exploring multiple identities and potential self-repertoires during life increases the resilience of personhood in the face of dementia, as the individual has a more varied and holistic definition of the self to inhabit.

Kitwood also argues that we are innately sacred and unique beings and that can never be threatened by the onset of disease.[15] If we can come into contact with this inherent concept of self, through any means, religious or otherwise, during life, then we can remain resilient. We have also to be prepared to participate in the joint construction of new selves, as suggested by Sabat and Harré.[10] Although some identities may be threatened by dementia, others may reveal themselves. We must be open to these new selves, in any setting, such as the reinvention of the previous high-functioning barrister as a kind person who takes care in opening the door at the day centre, or helping another resident eat at the nursing home. It is a different social role to be sure, to be now known as that kind person who always opens the door, rather than a barrister in court. But that perception is an identity in the minds of others. It is curious that whilst new parents revel in the most elemental interactions between their children at a childcare centre, the same elemental interactions between nursing home residents are rarely viewed with the same creativity and acceptance.

Whilst these interactions may be different from those traditionally valued by cognitively intact adults, they are no less meaningful. Often the main fear expressed regarding dementia is a life without meaning, or a living death. But there is always meaning when two people interact, verbally or non-verbally, with or without dementia. We must ask ourselves what do we really value and who are we really? Are we defined by our achievements, credentials and possessions, or by our compassionate, kind and simple interactions with family and other people? Whilst intellect and achievement undoubtedly help define us, we have other attributes and a spirituality that makes us who we are. If we can learn to appreciate the holistic nature of ourselves that encompasses the intellectual, emotional and the spiritual, we can be reassured that dementia can never threaten our true 'selves'.

Reinforcing efforts at self-maintenance

Recognising that identity is not a static quantity and that it changes over a life is also a useful concept in maintaining personhood. PwD often work hard to maintain identity when interacting with others after the onset of their dementia; for example, some research has shown that responses such as humour when confronted with a memory difficulty by others do not necessarily imply denial, they can be an active attempt to assert one's self and maintain a sense of control in a difficult situation.[17]

Furthermore, social interaction is needed as a sounding board so that PwD have an opportunity to try out new and old ways of communicating with others. It is well known that feeling isolated can be as toxic to one's health as smoking 20 cigarettes a day during life.[18] I would suspect that for PwD, being socially isolated is even more dangerous, as the social self has little opportunity for expression in a social vacuum. Even small, seemingly inconsequential interactions with others have powerful effects, not only on the brain, but also the soul.

I often explain to people in the memory clinic that it is very natural to want to avoid social activities if people become concerned about their social 'performance' due to memory or language difficulties. However, this is when these activities are needed most. And most people appraise their social performance more critically than others do, and there is rarely any expectation that PwD are expected to interact in any particular way. Just being with others is important. Constantly providing witty anecdotes less so.

How can PwD be helped to maintain their sense of identity and themselves? The reality is that many are surrounded by people who already do this intuitively. Even the smallest interaction with others is an opportunity to affirm, or negate, the other individual. The effects of these interactions accrue on a daily basis to provide a prevailing sense of social confirmation or negation, and also precise evidence of whether dementia will or will not undermine the person socially. We routinely witness both, even within the artificial confines of the memory clinic, and it is fairly normal that both should occur whilst people surrounding a PwD adjust to a diagnosis of dementia.

Here, the differing views of care of dementia, flagged by Kitwood, come into play and focus. At the initial point of diagnosis, there will be the opposing considerations of providing enough information to the clinician to support or disconfirm the diagnosis. As a doctor, I rely on collateral from family regarding the chronology of a cognitive impairment to diagnose a dementia. It is not uncommon for the PwD to have incomplete insight into the history of his/her memory disturbance. Immediately, there is a difficult line to tread. How do you obtain important information without appearing to negate or override the history of the person that it relates to?

I think transparency, acknowledgement and inclusion are the key at this early point – frequently explaining why the information is being sought, recognising that the process of being spoken about may be very strange. Explaining what the information means and what it doesn't. How it is about hearing and making sense of the story, and later explaining what dementia is and what it isn't. It is important that the person in question remains at the centre of the process. Often a well-intended relative will request to speak to me separately, to relay information that they feel will be distressing or difficult to hear, but I believe strongly that this needs to be relayed in front of the person being examined, otherwise an odd dynamic of being overridden and side-lined can establish itself.

Safeguarding all components of the self

How can others help in supporting the identity of those with dementia? The 'evidence-based' strategies mentioned above should come as no surprise. Listening to people's stories and their narratives; engaging people individually in meaningful activity; listening and looking carefully for communication that may not be as immediately obvious as previously; attending to someone at the end of their lives as consciously as we do for those as the beginning. None of these approaches is rocket science, and they are intuitive for many people as these are social responses that are innate to being human and caring. But, time and patience are not always in unlimited supply and it is important for carers not to be too hard on themselves for not always being person-centred.

Rather than focusing on one aspect of identity, why not guard all components of self? The first trap to avoid is an incorrect focus on memory, and for people to know that identity and personhood do not solely rely on this. Also for a greater awareness that science and theory exist that say we are more than our memories – that the self is expressed in many ways: in our relationships, in our life roles, in our interactions with others; that the self is held in the body, not just the mind; that the self does not need words to express itself; that the self can reveal itself in the smallest encounters with others; that most research into the self in dementia suggests that at least some aspects of the self remain in dementia, particularly the ability to use 'I', and to meaningfully communicate with others with or without words, and to occupy roles in relation to others.[8] All this should come as a comfort to those with dementia.

I have summarised some of these ideas earlier in the chapter, but they cannot be overstated enough in relation to dementia. Again, I think the majority of people affected by the condition intuitively believe many of these concepts about the self, but relaying them explicitly can do much to override the fear of dementia as a purely degenerative disease of the brain, the mind and the self.

Risk versus the self

In a medical setting, what is most important in self-hood maintenance is the explicit recognition that there is a tendency to prioritise other concepts instead. Risk is the main culprit. The most common scenario where this happens is when paid care is recommended to address a perceived care need. Typically, a PwD may not be attending to personal care as well as he/she has done previously. But, there is often a fierce sense of independence and a reluctance to accept a paid carer into the home.

Here again, a dialectical response to competing concerns regarding risk and the individual's wishes and preferences is needed. Accepting care may represent an affront to independent aspects of the self, such as self-reliance, autonomy and often a fear of becoming a burden on loved ones. In this situation, two extreme responses could be contemplated. One would be to prioritise and minimise risks of self-neglect through the installation of a comprehensive care package in the home or an enforced move to a residential home with 24-hour care. On the other hand, if individual autonomy is prioritised, then the wish not to have any care is respected and care needs are ignored.

Fortunately, there is a middle ground that can be explored to satisfy the competing demands of self-autonomy and risk. Care levels and input can be arranged at different levels. When this is delivered by nuanced and person-centred carers, who are very aware of the individual's strong sense of autonomy, care can be delivered creatively, respectfully and non-intrusively. I think it is useful to point out that when there is an objection to 'a carer coming into the home', this objection often disappears when the abstract concept of carer is replaced with 'Jill' or 'Sam' who visits regularly and forms a social connection. Bonds quickly form and social interactions beyond the care process naturally occur, bolstering a sense of self and appeasing previous overarching catastrophic predictions regarding threat to autonomy.

A vivid example of the friction between risk and self that comes to mind and serves as a reminder of how we need to be open to creative attempts to maintain the self, concerns a war veteran with dementia. A retired war veteran had recently changed carers and during one interaction brandished an old war pistol at the new carer. The situation escalated quickly. The police were called, the offending weapon removed and the man became unsettled and agitated to the degree that anti-psychotic medication was administered and admission to a psychiatric ward was considered.

What had happened, however, was that the (non-functional) pistol was being shown to the new carer as an active attempt by the man to explain to his new carer that being a serviceman was an important part of his identity. The carer being new to the situation, and receiving no biographical information about his client from prior carers, had interpreted the pistol display as a potential example of aggression. The police had also unfortunately interpreted the encounter as an incident of concern and the pistol was removed to reduce risk. However, this unsettled the man further and the man's attempt to assert his identity with a new person backfired, having been labelled as risk. Although few episodes of the risk–self friction are this dramatic, it emphasises how one can trump the other in the absence of information. The pistol episode could have also been prevented if the encounter had been contextualised within the man's life story and personal narrative.

'Wandering' also deserves specific mention when considering the potential conflict between self-autonomy and perceived risk. Again, this is most easily demonstrated through anecdote. A lady in her 80s, with established dementia, began to 'wander'. Her sons were so concerned that someone stayed to supervise her each night. On further questioning of the family, it became clear that her 'wandering' was both infrequent and purposeful. Over the preceding three months, she had woken on two occasions in the early morning, and thinking it was later, had walked to the local shop about a mile away to buy a local paper. On both occasions, she was found waiting patiently for the shop to open, without apparent distress or concern. It was also known that previously she and her husband (now deceased) had owned a newsagent shop for 20 years and she had taken ownership of paper delivery.

Whilst her family thought that her 'wandering' could represent an active attempt to maintain part of a previous occupational identity, they were too concerned by the risk associated with this behaviour, such as pedestrian safety and also hypothermia when the winter arrived. Whilst other families I have encountered were happier to accept incidents of 'wandering', and mitigated associated risks such as ensuring coats were worn, it can be difficult for a family to accept that an active attempt to maintain one's sense of purpose in dementia can be risky. In an ideal situation, the environment could be improved to mitigate risks, meaning that PwD could wander as they chose. The term 'wandering' has also been questioned as to whether it is helpful, as it implies a zombie-like trance rather than a purposeful activity.[19] In many cases, wandering is meaningful in some way.

The role of 'expert families' in preserving the self

I am often impressed by the numerous families who have intuitively wrestled with the concept of self in dementia and found a way through. An example was a man with a dementia that profoundly affected his ability to speak. He previously owned a computer business and was a keen tennis player. His family used both of these roles and aspects of his identity creatively in response to other problems. An example was his personal care. He was reluctant to change his clothes each day and was resistant when this issue was forced. However, he still played tennis with his children several times a week and he happily changed to new clothes when these were offered before he played a game, as he was previously used to changing before playing.

He also had a tendency to 'wander', and would walk several miles to his old business and other computer stores attempting to help. This was managed on several fronts. The police dealing with his occasional unwanted help at shops knew his background and what this behaviour represented. When these episodes occurred, shop owners were given some explanatory background and he was taken home with a minimum of fuss. Old computers were also placed in a garage so he had a 'shop' to tinker in at home, rather than walking back to his old one.

Whilst this man's refusal to change clothes and wandering to computer shops could have had many different outcomes, the family's intuitive sense of their father allowed a nuanced and person-centred solution to difficulty.

Ultimately, we need more research to understand how PwD experience a sense of themselves and relate to others whilst they navigate the condition. These understandings can then be used to help develop more person-centred interventions. Whilst these are developed, we need to keep the person in mind and adopt a curious and creative approach to dementia. Maintaining social interactions, being open to our multiple definitions of the self, being mindful of threats to the self and prioritising the self above other considerations, such as risk, may all help in preserving the individual in the face of dementia.

II. (MARY)

Noel has written so extensively and so eloquently on this subject that I have little to add except from a personal perspective. The discussion of 'personhood' in dementia has been covered at length by many writers but, in my experience, it is a subject less often referred to by the people most nearly concerned – that is PwD and their carers and families. If asked, most carers will state that the person they care for is still very much the same character, although some of the character traits have become more obvious or emphasised – and research tends to bear out this opinion.[20]

A great deal of work has been and is being done to give those whose memories are seen to be failing an 'anchor', in the form of life story work or the variously named 'life boxes', and many elderly people enjoy the idea of creating their life story. I only question whether it is as necessary as some advocates suggest. During life, we evolve and change as a person. The person we are at age 60 is not the same as the person we were at age six and the things we enjoy and occupy ourselves with change too. Our character may not have changed, but the things we enjoy or do may have. Our life with dementia may involve enjoyment of many things which we would not have contemplated doing prior to cognitive problems arising.

Noel is right to state that we need more research to understand how 'PwD experience a sense of themselves and relate to others whilst they navigate the condition'. In my everyday contact with PwD, and with those who care for them, I most often hear a plea that the community accept those with dementia for what they are now in the present. A discussion at a dementia café came to this conclusion recently: 'It would be nice if we could just feel that we are who we are and live normally – why does everyone have to define us by the illness of dementia?'

REFERENCES

1. Merriam-Webster Online Dictionary. *Self.* https://www.merriam-webster.com/dictionary/self (accessed 26 June 2017).

2. Wikipedia. *Self.* https://en.wikipedia.org/wiki/Self (accessed 26 June 2017).

3. Rapaport D. *Emotions and Memory.* Baltimore: Williams & Wilkins; 1942.

4. Conway MA. Memory and the self. *Journal of Memory and Language* 2005; 53(4): 594-628.

5. Touhy TA. Dementia, personhood, and nursing: learning from a nursing situation. *Nursing Science Quarterly* 2004; 17(1): 43-9.

6. Doyle PJ, Rubinstein RL. Person-centered dementia care and the cultural matrix of othering. *Gerontologist* 2014 Dec; 54(6): 952-63.

7. Beard RL, Neary TM. Making sense of nonsense: experiences of mild cognitive impairment. *Sociology of Health & Illness* 2013; 35(1): 130-46.

8. Caddell LS, Clare L. The impact of dementia on self and identity: A systematic review. *Clinical Psychology Review* 2010; 30(1): 113-26.

9. Marks D. Models of disability. *Disability and Rehabilitation* 1997; 19(3): 85-91.

10. Sabat SR, Harré R. The construction and deconstruction of self in Alzheimer's disease. *Ageing and Society* 1992; 12(04): 443-61.

11. Kitwood T. The dialectics of dementia: with particular reference to Alzheimer's disease. *Ageing and Society* 1990; 10(02): 177-96.

12. Kontos PC. Ethnographic reflections on selfhood, embodiment and Alzheimer's disease. *Ageing and Society* 2004; 24(6): 829-49.

13. Kontos P. Musical embodiment, selfhood, and dementia. In: Hydén LC, Lindemann H, Brockmeier J (eds) *Beyond Loss: Dementia, Identity, Personhood.* Oxford: Oxford University Press; 2014: 107-19.

14. Perry J. Expanding the dialogue on dementia: (Re)positioning diagnosis and narrative. *Canadian Journal of Nursing Research* 2005; 37(2): 166-80.

15. Kitwood T. Dementia reconsidered: the person comes first. In: Katz J, Peace S, Spurr S (eds) *Adult Lives: A Life Course Perspective.* Bristol: Policy Press; 2011: 89.

16. McKeown J, Clarke A, Ingleton C, Ryan T, Repper J. The use of life

story work with people with dementia to enhance person-centred care. *International Journal of Older People Nursing* 2010; 5(2): 148-58.

17. Saunders PA. 'My brain's on strike': The construction of identity through memory accounts by dementia patients. *Research on Aging* 1998; 20(1): 65-90.

18. Cacioppo JT, Cacioppo S. Social relationships and health: The toxic effects of perceived social isolation. *Social and personality psychology compass* 2014; 8(2): 58-72.

19. Behuniak SM. The living dead? The construction of people with Alzheimer's disease as zombies. *Ageing and Society* 2011; 31(01): 70-92.

20. Nicholas H et al. Are abnormal premorbid personality traits a marker for Alzheimer's Disease? A case controlled study. *International Journal of Geriatric Psychiatry* 2010; 25(4): 345-351.

21. Genova L. *Still Alice*. London: Simon & Schuster UK, Reissue edition; 2012.

22. *Alive Inside*. [YouTube film] added by Alive Inside Foundation 2012. https://www.youtube.com/watch?v=Hlm0Qd4mP-I (accessed 22 July 2017).

Chapter 5

Dementia as a cognitive disability

Summary

- Purely medical models of disability have been criticised for locating disability solely in the affected individual.

- A social model of disability argues that disability is not an inevitable consequence of impairment if the environment steps up to support the individual.

- A cognitive disability model focuses on residual skill, rather than deficit, and explicitly describes strategies to maintain function and 're-able' the individual.

- Using a social model of cognitive disability in dementia highlights how current health and social care policy actively disables those with a cognitive impairment.

- A social model of cognitive disability and a biomedical model of dementia are not mutually exclusive and can be used together in a complementary way.

- Dementia can usefully be defined as a disability rather than an impairment; there are advantages and disadvantages to this approach.

- We can benefit by looking at the approaches that other countries, such as the Netherlands, have taken to care for people with dementia.

- A supportive environment can make a dramatic difference to how someone copes with a diagnosis of dementia.

- A supportive environment is one that is as low in stress as possible and also safe and stimulating.

- Nidotherapy is a form of mental health therapy which can be adapted to help those with dementia.

I. (NOEL)
What can the disability model offer dementia?

One of the aims of this book is to introduce the reader to alternative conceptualisations of dementia. In this chapter, Mary and I explore how people with dementia (PwD) might benefit from dementia being thought of as a cognitive disability rather than as a brain disease, as is usual. To do this, we first examine what disability is, then explore the notion of cognitive disability, and the advantages and disadvantages of viewing dementia in this way. We do this by examining several models of disability that have advanced the cause of the disability movement over the last few decades, and improved the lives of people living with disabilities. Lastly, we look at how the model of a cognitive disability can be used successfully alongside other frameworks of dementia in a meaningful and helpful way to help mitigate disability associated with dementia.

Disability definitions

In order to examine the concept of cognitive disability, the term 'disability' needs to be defined. Defining disability can be problematic as it arises not just from individual factors such as disease or an impairment, but also from the environment's inability to accommodate an impairment. Medical models of disability tend to locate the cause of disability in the individual, usually arising from some disease or biological impairment. An example is the eye condition macular degeneration, which causes visual impairment and a subsequent disability. In contrast, social models of disability argue that whilst impairments have biological origins, it is the environmental conditions in society that create or negate the resultant disability. An often-cited definition of disability from the World Health Organization incorporates both medical and social models, and emphasises that disability results from the interaction of both individual and societal factors:

> Disabilities is an umbrella term, covering impairments, activity limitations, and participation restrictions. An impairment is a problem in body function or structure; an activity limitation is a difficulty encountered by an individual in executing a task or action; while a participation restriction is a problem experienced by an individual in involvement in life situations.
>
> Disability is thus not just a health problem. It is a complex phenomenon, reflecting the interaction between features of a person's body and features of the society in which he or she lives. Overcoming the difficulties faced by people with disabilities requires interventions to remove environmental and social barriers.[1]

If disability is defined in this way, then the difference between impairment and disability is highlighted and, in particular, a disability is not an inevitable consequence of an impairment if the environment steps up to support the individual with any given impairment. This also is the case with cognitive impairment, where a supportive environment and other social structures can mitigate the effect of a cognitive disability. Before looking at this more closely, I will examine different models of disability to explore ways in which 'cognitive disability' may be a useful construct in dementia.

Disability models

Medical model of disability

As already introduced, there are different models of disability. The traditional medical model tends to focus on the individual and how a biological deficit or disease process can result in a personal disability. The natural consequence of this perspective is that it activates a medical approach whereby any efforts to assist the individual to live with his/her disability, through rehabilitation or assistive aids, is organised around a medical diagnosis. Health and social care policy makers have also made strategic decisions regarding health and care planning based on medicalised definitions of disability, such as that in the *International Classification of Impairments, Disabilities and Handicaps (ICIDH)*.[2]

This also occurs with cognitive impairment and dementia. Projections of the increasing prevalence of dementia are often cited as a 'dementia epidemic', in order to mobilise politicians and health and social care policy makers. Although an increasing rate of dementia and cognitive impairment is to be expected in any ageing population, projections of the increasing dementia prevalence say little about the needs of this cognitively impaired population, and, in particular, the nature of cognitive disability for most within this group. Who will remain at home? Who will require residential care? What supports are needed to keep this group healthy? What supports do family and other carers need to maintain networks of support? What policy or environmental changes could be employed to keep the majority of PwD independent for as long as possible?

Instead, health and social care policy makers remain focused on medical aspects of dementia care such as the prescription of memory-enhancing drugs, anti-psychotics and care costs. Using a cognitive disability model rather than viewing dementia as an epidemic of neurodegenerative disease would recognise the diversity of (dis)abilities of PwD and shift the policy debate about dementia from disease and death to a positive discourse around maintaining abilities and independence.

Medical models of disability have been criticised for locating disability purely in the affected individual. This then creates an imperative to make people with disabilities fit into mainstream society rather than making the social environment accessible for all. The medical model has also been criticised for pathologising impairment and ignoring the fact that disability is a natural state for most people at some point during their lives.[3] The medical model of disability also ignores how social structures and policy can exclude people with physical impairments, by focusing on the biological causes of impairment.[4]

Social models of disability

In contrast to this, social models of disability highlight environmental and social factors as maintainers of disability. This displaces the idea that disabilities are inevitable consequences of biological impairment, and suggests that disabilities are instead the consequence of an oppressive social environment that only serves the able-bodied. This perspective shifts the focus to consideration of how social policy and the physical environment need to be changed to be more facilitative for people with disabilities. It is argued that the social model of disability has evolved out of the disability movement's advocacy for citizenship, rights and independence for disabled people.[3] This has in turn 'successfully politicised social and physical space by drawing attention to the ways in which dominant, non-disabled values and practices constitute vast tracts of space as no-go-areas'.[4]

Dementia can benefit from the approach contained within the social disability model. Rather than dementia being narrowly viewed as a brain pathology in an individual that might eventually be cured, or at least controlled with a cognitive enhancer or anti-amyloid agent, the social disability model asks questions about how our day-to-day environment could be made more user-friendly for those with cognitive impairment. It also poses questions about aspects of social policy that discriminate against those with cognitive impairments, covertly preventing their active engagement with greater society. When applied to dementia, the social model of disability challenges the traditional medical view that disability arises purely as a result of an individual's deficit, rather than from socially created barriers to full participation and citizenship.[4]

Affirmative social model of disability

There are differing social models of disability which have potential utility in thinking about dementia. One is the affirmative model of disability. This is defined by Swain and French as 'a non-tragic view of disability and impairment which encompasses positive social identities, both individual and collective, for disabled people grounded in the … life experience of being impaired and disabled'.[5] Can this affirmative model be used in dementia, even though the cognitive impairment in dementia is progressive?

There are many reasons why an affirmative model could be meaningfully applied in dementia. The rising prevalence of older adult dementia is a potent example of humans successfully living longer and this new reality should in itself be affirmed, not denied. On a more personal level, I often say to people who comment that my professional life as a dementia doctor must be depressing, that some of the happiest people I meet have dementia, and that whilst dementia is a challenging family and personal event, it often brings out the best in people – in particular, the robustness of the human spirit in navigating loss and difficulty with kindness, love and care.

I do not deny the tragic aspects of dementia, but I do challenge the often-prevalent notion that all aspects of dementia are tragic. Dementia, like any illness, is also a social experience, and parts of this experience are inherently positive, irrespective of the prognosis of the underlying 'condition'. An affirmative and non-tragic model of cognitive disability recognises this reality and goes some way to challenge the 'rhetoric of loss' that surrounds dementia and cognitive impairment, specifically that the future is lost and there is only a past.

Cognitive disability models

What do we mean by 'cognitive disability'? Using the aforementioned disability definition, a cognitive disability encompasses any cognitive impairment that results in an individual's difficulty to execute actions or participate in life due to the impairment. Like disability in general, it will reflect the interaction between intrinsic factors, the environment and social barriers. Although a mild cognitive impairment (MCI) is distinguished from dementia by preserved function, a cognitive disability considers impairment in broader terms as anything that precludes full engagement with society compared with someone else who is more cognitively 'abled'. Although the concept of cognitive disability is not used explicitly by the medical profession when considering dementia, it is used more widely by other health professionals such as neuro-psychologists and occupational therapists, and when considering rehabilitation in traumatic or post-stroke cognitive impairment.

An example of a cognitive disability model is one developed in the 1960s by Claudia Allen et al. This model assesses cognitive function within a continuum of ability and aims to:

> ... promote a person's 'best ability to function' and allow people to live in the least restrictive environment where they are guided in occupational-based interventions at the level of activity demands, performance skills, and occupations based on the Occupational Therapy Practice Framework and in line with the WHO *International Classification of Function (ICF).*[6]

Advantages of using a cognitive disability approach in dementia

The advantage of the cognitive disability conceptual model is that it focuses on residual skill, rather than just deficit, and explicitly describes strategies to maintain function.[7] Some neuropsychologists, who are trained in this approach and who work within memory clinics and make regular neuropsychometric assessments of PwD, will make similar recommendations centred around the maintenance of life skills and daily function. However, these reports are specialised and require considerable time to compile, in comparison with purely diagnostic neuropsychometric reports that aim to just make a diagnosis of dementia.

Access to neuropsychometry with a rehabilitative focus, conducted by a neuropsychologist familiar with a cognitive disability model, is very limited, as it a service not prioritised by health commissioners in the current Tory era of austerity. It may also be that rehabilitation of cognitive disability in the context of dementia is viewed as difficult and ultimately pointless. This is despite the possibility of 'rementia' with appropriate guidance and support for PwD and their carers.[8]

Adopting a cognitive disability model in dementia recognises the potential for improvement despite the progressive nature of the condition, which is rarely linear in its decline. It also shares an underlying optimism with the social affirmative model of disability, in that disability accords an opportunity to demonstrate individual resilience and creativity in the face of biological obstacles and challenge. Investing in a cognitive disability model of dementia and the more routine application of rehabilitative neuropsychometry is also a potent demonstration that society is willing to invest in increasing the potential of PwD, which is at the centre of social models of disability. If using a social model of disability in dementia activates public interest, policy debate and an advocacy platform on the issue, then this is a success in its own right.

What are the other advantages of using a cognitive disability model when viewing dementia?

To begin with, it immediately shifts the focus of discourse on dementia away from a reductionist and nihilistic biomedical account of an individual's brain pathology and resultant deficits, to something inherently more positive and helpful. That is, it focuses on what can be done on a social and environmental level to 're-able' the individual to engage meaningfully with society.

Using the lens of a social disability model in dementia can also help broaden society's current narrow view of dementia, and lessen its myopic focus on 'finding a cure'. Instead, there could be an examination of how current health and social care policy and law actively disable those with a cognitive impairment and dementia. Gabel and Peters remind us that disabling social policy is only visible by its effects.[9] Some examples include:

• Existing hospital targets, such as the four-hour waiting rule in Accident and Emergency, which means that people with cognitive impairments often change ward environment several times within a 24-hour period. This avoids financial penalties for the hospital but increases disorientation for the individual and makes continuity of care more difficult.

- The increasing privatisation of the social care sector, and cost pressures on private providers, leading to minimal carer staffing of residential homes and an increasing focus on meeting basic and instrumental need, rather than facilitating any positive social exchanges for PwD.

- A lack of discourse about positive risk-taking to maximise autonomy, combined with the effects of the Mental Capacity Act 2005, is leading to record numbers of PwD having their deprivation of liberty being legally sanctioned, rather than exploring how their liberty could be maximised through environmental change. Current national 'Deprivation of liberty safeguards' are now routinely used by private nursing home providers to avoid risk or criticism from external regulators, in preference to local informal arrangements with families that balance autonomy and risk.

Other advantages of applying a cognitive disability model to dementia assessment and care include a greater focus on support post-diagnosis, rather than just diagnosis itself. Currently, in the UK there has been a politicised emphasis on increasing the diagnosis rate in dementia. Diagnosis has been financially incentivised in acute hospitals which are very challenging places to assess anyone's memory. This has meant that resources of Community Mental Health Teams have been shifted to diagnosis rather than support of people affected by mild cognitive impairment and dementia.

Post-diagnostic support has also been increasingly shunted into the voluntary 'third' sector, which suffers from patchy funding, often spread very thinly. On the ground, this means that it can be difficult for PwD and the cognitively impaired to access advice or support about how best to live with the condition. Instead, PwD are medicalised and labelled from the outset as victims of dementia. If they are lucky, they will be offered cognitive enhancers for the condition (which have modest effects at best), and be referred for a care needs assessment from the local authority – which is usually unable to offer any paid support unless strict financial criteria are met. This traditional post-diagnostic trajectory rarely offers any neuropsychological assessment, which highlights cognitive strengths as well as weaknesses. Nor is there routine domiciliary occupational therapy input, whereby the home environment can be inspected and modified in order to maximise function and potential to live at home independently.

Whilst we continue to focus on the elusive 'cure just around the corner', with the alluring prospect of disease-modifying anti-amyloid agents, this once again focuses the attention regarding dementia on the individual's pathology, rather than on societal and environmental processes that could be changed to make the daily lives of the cognitively impaired easier. Instead of seeing the increasing prevalence of cognitive disability in our ageing society as a challenge, we could view it as an opportunity to make our world more accessible for all, rather than continuing to pathologise and disable those with cognitive impairment. Marks reminds us that:

> … we need to rethink our culture, institutions and relationships in order to create a more inclusive society which can tolerate a higher degree of differences. Disability studies become the analysis not of disabled people, but the study of the way in which we think and live in society.[3]

Given that cognitive impairment and disability will become an increasing reality for many people, a cognitive disability model of dementia affords an opportunity to examine how society can empower individuals of all cognitive abilities, not just those with dementia, but also children and those with traumatic brain injury and learning disabilities. Nussbaum eloquently surmises that 'people with cognitive disabilities are equal citizens, and the law ought to show respect for them as full equals'.[10]

Disadvantages of a cognitive disability approach in dementia

What is the counter argument for pursuing a cognitive disability model in dementia? There is always a danger in following any one model religiously to the exclusion of all others. The social model of disability is no different, and applied in its purest form is too polarising and dismissive of the medical model. I have been deliberately provocative in my descriptions above of how medical processes can inadvertently disenfranchise, and disable, those with cognitive impairments through locating cognitive disability solely in the individual to the neglect of social and environmental processes. The opposite also holds. Proponents of incentivising dementia diagnoses argue that without a diagnosis there can be no post-diagnostic support. And even though cognitive enhancers have modest effects, there is no doubt that the prescription of these medications in medical memory clinic settings has been instrumental in countering the pervasive therapeutic nihilism that previously existed in dementia care.

It may also be difficult for many to apply the model of cognitive disability in the setting of a progressive and terminal condition like dementia. Even though the course and prognosis can vary widely, dementia often results in death. Hence a palliative approach, rather than a rehabilitative one centred on a disability model, may be preferred, particularly if the diagnosis is made late. The reality is that a palliative approach centred on care and amelioration of distress, and rehabilitation for cognitive disability, are not mutually exclusive. Any caring and empathic social interaction between a PwD and a carer is likely to have reassuring and 'rementing' qualities.

Both the social disability and biomedical models of dementia, if pursued in extremis, can create unhealthy splits between the mind, body and society. Neither on its own can fully account for both ability and disability in dementia. Hughes and Paterson comment that both models treat the body as:

> ... a pre-social, inert, physical object, as discrete, palpable and separate from the self. The definition of impairment proposed by the social model of disability recapitulates the biomedical 'faulty machine' model of the body.[4]

They go on to say that:

> ... the social model of disability proposes an untenable separation between body and culture, impairment and disability. While this has been of enormous value in establishing a radical politics of disability, the Cartesianised subject that it produces sits very uneasily in the contemporary world.[4]

Using a cognitive disability approach alongside other models

The ultimate aim of this chapter is not to suggest that the medical model of dementia should be abandoned in favour of a cognitive disability model, social or otherwise. Instead I hope to have argued a central tenet of this whole book – that dementia can benefit from varied viewpoints from several models that are not mutually exclusive in their application. It is not either/or. Differing models such as a biomedical and a social disability model can be used in harmony with each other. In fact, this confluence of theory occurs in the day-to-day practice of any multi-disciplinary team working with PwD. Team membership benefits from a number of people from different traditions, including doctors, social workers, nurses, occupational therapists and psychologists, working together. Biomedical, psychological and social factors are all examined as a consequence.

What can be questioned, however, is the traditional dominance of the biomedical model in dementia, such that medicine assumes ownership of the condition and people affected by it. Alternative approaches contained within other paradigms should receive equal attention and recognition. Marks explains that:

> ... a balanced analysis of disability looks not only at the disabled individual, but also at the disabling environment. We should not see impairment as 'fundamental', but rather as one factor in the social construction of disability. It is important to add that a social analysis does not rule out medical or prosthetic interventions which may be appropriate and desirable. However, it does reject the notion that prevention or cure of disability is a panacea.[3]

If the use of the word 'disability' is prefaced with 'cognitive' in Marks' comments, then the vision of how more holistic understandings of dementia, using a medical and a social disability model of cognitive impairment together, can be appreciated. Given that the world's population is ageing and cognitive disability will be an increasing reality for many, perhaps affecting a third of people at some stage of their life, future societies will have no choice but to adopt this ideal to ensure ongoing citizenship of all its members.

Go Dutch?

Holland is probably one the best countries in the world at changing the physical environment to reduce the likelihood of disability in people with impairments. There are so many creative schemes being pursued it is difficult to know where to begin, but several remarkable endeavours spring to mind. One example is that of the 'dementia village' where there are carefully planned and supported environments where the effects of a cognitive disability are minimised. These villages are safe places where PwD can live rewarding and fulfilling lives, helped by a large number of volunteers and professionals who adopt roles as friends rather than supervisory clinicians.[11]

Another creative programme is a scheme where students can live rent free in nursing homes in exchange for some volunteer work and spending time with the local residents.[12] This co-resident exchange programme combats the social isolation and loneliness that exists in nursing homes and kills residents prematurely. This kind of 'blue sky' thinking is the way forward for people to reduce cognitive disability in those with cognitive impairments through creative means. Although I think these approaches are the future in dementia care, they are unlikely to find wide application in the UK. This is due to cost in staffing and infrastructure and the unlikelihood that reducing cognitive disability will ever become a policy priority in dementia care.

II. (MARY)

It is important to realise that everyday living is stressful for people who have a cognitive impairment. The actions that we take to maintain our existence each day, such as washing, dressing, preparing food, keeping the environment clean and hygienic, shopping and so on, may sometimes seem like a chore especially if we are tired or unwell, but they do not generally overtax us. People with dementia, however, can find these actions of daily living (ADLs) difficult to cope with even when they are not tired, unwell or overstressed. When stressed by any untoward event, by a change in routine, or through being challenged by a physical infection, simple ADLs become an insurmountable obstacle.

In this situation, the PwD either 'gives up' entirely and becomes effectively helpless or gets angry and frustrated and perhaps reacts aggressively. Carers and family members sometimes become quite annoyed when the person they care for is unable to cope with a simple action which they have managed before. They may think that the PwD is being deliberately awkward and obstructive. Even if they can see the reason for the temporary difficulty, they are likely to become impatient and stressed.

The best environment for someone with dementia: the three 'S's

- First, it is important that the environment is *supportive*. Life does not always run smoothly and those of us who still have plentiful cognitive reserves learn to cope with that fact. We reason with ourselves when we get bad tempered – the weather is bad, the traffic is heavy, the car has developed a fault, the dishwasher needs repairing, an important appointment has been cancelled – these are the things which have led to our feeling upset. We deal with life's problems and overcome the obstacles and 'come out the other side' and life resumes its smooth pleasant aspect. Someone who has little cognitive reserve, for whom even following routine is difficult, will find any change or complication doubly difficult. People with dementia need support. They need support from those around them and they need a supportive environment, an environment which makes it easier for them to cope.

- Secondly, the environment should feel *safe*. Note that I am not saying here that the environment should *be* safe but that it should *feel* safe to the PwD. Naturally we should aim for a safe home environment – we should deal with risks and potential hazards in terms of preventing falls and other accidents and ensure that the PwD cannot unwittingly cause an accident due to a lack of sensible precautions, but in this chapter we are discussing reducing stress for PwD, and in that sense it is vital that the home and local environment *feel* safe.

- A common saying of PwD is 'I want to go home.' When I am training carers, I ask them to imagine why this is being said so frequently. They often suggest that it is connected with memory – that the person with dementia is remembering their old home from childhood days – their memory is slipping back to the past. But let us consider what the term 'home' means to most of us. It means a place where we feel relaxed and comfortable, where we do not have to make an effort or show a special face to the world, and above all, a place of safety. So when PwD say they want to go home they are most often expressing the fact that they do not feel either safe or comfortable. Some care homes have actually understood this and have an area of the building that they term the 'safe area' where people who are upset can be taken in order that they can feel comfortable and secure. Other residential homes may call this the 'quiet area', but it still has essentially the same meaning.

- Thirdly, the preferred environment for PwD should be *stimulating* to the senses and provide an opportunity for social interaction. At first sight, this may seem to conflict with the suggestion of a safe relaxing environment but the two are not mutually incompatible. Carers often complain that the PwD does nothing but fall asleep when they are at home. The fact is that without stimulation any of us may become bored and doze off. How often has this happened to you whilst watching a boring TV programme? People with dementia are frequently bored because many of the occupations with which they passed the time previously are now closed to them. Boredom can lead to difficult behaviour and restlessness, but often it just results in sleepiness.

Nidotherapy

This form of therapy was developed initially as an approach to treating people with long-term, treatment-resistant mental problems. Peter Tyrer, author of *Nidotherapy: Harmonising the Environment with the Patient* writes that:

> ... nidotherapy is introduced ... to change the environment to create better adaptation in however slight a degree to the mental state conditions.[13]

His book suggests that:

> ... [for the persistently mentally ill] we should abandon the strategy of getting them to compete with others who are conventionally more fortunate and better able to compete, and instead attempt to match their special strengths with environments that suit them and which are not troubled by their weaknesses.[3]

If we are to view dementia as a cognitive disability rather than a terminal 'illness', then making adjustments to the environment of a PwD makes perfect sense, and the nidotherapy approach fits perfectly with this concept. Nidotherapy (the term originates from the Latin word for nest), aims to listen to what the 'patient' is saying about his/her environment and how this affects him or her. It takes the person's wishes seriously. Instead of trying to change the person to fit in better with the environment, the aim is to change the environment to better fit the person. From the point of view of helping a PwD this is quite a dramatic suggestion. Most therapy and intervention in dementia are aimed at helping the person who has the cognitive difficulty to fit into the world as we see it.

How would nidotherapy work in practice in dementia?

Nidotherapy fits exceptionally well with the three 'S's of the best environment for a PwD (supportive, safe, stimulating). Implementing and monitoring what is called a 'nido-pathway' may be a little different when applied to dementia rather than to mental health, but a care supporter can still analyse the environment, elicit the wishes of the PwD and formulate suggestions for change.

This discussion about environment does not only apply to the immediate (i.e. home) environment. It may be that changes to the wider environment can have significant effects on the wellbeing of the PwD. For example, the local neighbourhood may be a fearful and confusing place to someone with a cognitive impairment. Factors worth considering: are all the houses in the street similar in design? Does this make it difficult for the PwD to find his/her home after walking out? Are there a confusing number of routes to reach the house or street – perhaps footpaths or shortcuts rather than direct street walking access? Are the neighbours hostile and unfriendly? Does this make walking out fraught with anxiety for someone who might mistake the right route or the correct front door?

We can take this concept farther and consider more far-flung environments. Are places which the PwD visits frequently (local shop/club/dog-walking routes) too difficult to negotiate, or too brightly patterned for someone with visual problems, or too unfriendly in terms of those that might be encountered there?

Dementia is a problem for all of society, but this is still little recognised. Most public places are now 'accessible' in terms of physical disability with level paths, ramps for wheeled access, better signage, bigger parking spaces and so on. Society should now consider making changes to improve accessibility for those with the cognitive disability we call dementia. Such changes might include material factors such as street signs, clear demarcation of different areas and well-defined entrances and exits, but they should also include the vital human factor. People with dementia need support from other humans – assistive technology can be helpful in a limited way but social interaction is what slows the slide into helplessness. Just as the public have been educated to recognise the rights and needs of those with a physical disability, so the rights and needs of those with a cognitive disability need now to be addressed in our neighbourhoods and public places.

REFERENCES

1. World Health Organization. *Disabilities*. http://www.who.int/topics/disabilities/en/ (accessed 27 June 2017).

2. World Health Organization. *International Classification of Impairments, Disabilities and Handicaps: A Manual of Classification Relating to the Consequences of Disease*. Geneva: WHO; 1980.

3. Marks D. Models of disability. *Disability and Rehabilitation* 1997; 19(3): 85-91.

4. Hughes B, Paterson K. The social model of disability and the disappearing body: Towards a sociology of impairment. *Disability &*

Society 1997; 12(3): 325-40.

5. Swain J, French S. Towards an affirmation model of disability. *Disability & Society* 2000; 15(4): 569-82.

6. Allen C, Austin S, David S, et al. *Manual for the Allen Cognitive Level Screen-5 (ACLS-5) and Large Allen Cognitive Level Screen-5 (LACLS-5)*. Camarillo, CA: ACLS and LACLS Committee; 2007.

7. Allen CK. Occupational therapy: Functional assessment of the severity of mental disorders. *Psychiatric Services* 1988; 39(2): 140-42.

8. Kitwood T. Dementia reconsidered: the person comes first. In: Katz J, Peace S, Spurr S (eds) *Adult Lives: A Life Course Perspective*. Bristol: Policy Press; 2011: 89.

9. Gabel S, Peters S. Presage of a paradigm shift? Beyond the social model of disability toward resistance theories of disability. *Disability & Society* 2004; 19(6): 585-600.

10. Nussbaum M. The capabilities of people with cognitive disabilities. *Metaphilosophy* 2009; 40(3-4): 331-51. dor: 10/1111/j.1467-9973.2009.01606.x

11. Jenkins C, Smythe A. Reflections on a visit to a dementia care village. *Nursing Older People* 2013; 25(6): 14-19.

12. Ali A. Students move-in with residents in Dutch nursing home and help combat social isolation and depression among elderly. *The Independent* 20th July 2015. www.independent.co.uk/student/news/students-move-in-with-residents-in-Dutch-nursing-home-and-help-combat-social-isolation-and-10401882.html (Accessed 28 August 2017)

13. Tyrer P. *Nidotherapy: Harmonising the Environment with the Patient*. London: Royal College of Psychiatrists Publications; 2009.

Chapter 6

Caring in dementia

Summary

- There are many facets to the term 'care' in dementia; care ranges from gentle support to complete management of the actions of daily living.

- Care needs in dementia can be very complicated and carers' experience can vary considerably.

- The expert carer understands the personal demands of the carer role and sets realistic expectations of their own performance.

- Formal (paid) and informal (unpaid) carers can learn from each other's experiences and will naturally conflict at times.

- Although much has been written about carer burden, there are positive effects of caring.

- Some people choose to be a carer and some have the role thrust upon them; however, each has to carry out the role and many have little training or information about how to do this.

- Carers themselves need extra support to carry out their caring role.

- It can be difficult to think ahead and foresee how the caring role will change as dementia progresses.

- Professional carers are often exploited by their employers and have low status and pay; nevertheless they frequently give excellent care to their clients.

- Family carers are often ignored by society and left unsupported and stressed.

I. (NOEL)
What is care?

Care is an innate human process as fundamental to life as breathing. Being so intrinsic and automatic to our nature, it can be difficult to define. It means different things to different people. Some focus on assistance with the practicalities of daily life; others see care as keeping another in mind and being responsive to arising needs. Whilst many would not identify with being a carer, as this implies a dedicated role, most would hope they are caring to friends and family in need. Although care is a concept that pervades the entire human life span, the care of children has different meanings from adult care. Whilst caring well for dependent minors is revered as the best example of our humanity, receiving care as a dependent adult mostly has universally negative connotations. To be in receipt of care is to be dependent on others, to lose control and relinquish autonomy and freedom. And to have dementia *and* need care is often portrayed as a worst-case scenario in life. But dementia, as a life event, evokes our caring instincts and reconnects us to a fundamental part of ourselves. Invariably, when I tell someone what I do for a living, it is remarked how depressing my job must be. I answer that I feel quite privileged to bear witness to quite remarkable exchanges of care between people.

As the world's population ages and cognitive impairment, dementia and frailty all increase in prevalence, it is likely that the care of older adults will enter more open discussion. By 2020, in many European countries, almost one quarter of the population will be over 65. And, as we said earlier, the over-85 group is the fastest-growing demographic.[1] Although it remains unclear exactly how healthy this population will be, as discussed in previous chapters, care needs in the overall population are likely to increase. This is frequently referred to in the popular media as an 'economic time bomb', with the assumption that the increasing need for care only has negative economic consequences.[2] But whilst caring for an older adult brings unique challenges for the individual and care systems of the world, it also provides an opportunity. Providing good care for another person is a satisfying endeavour and can provide benefits as well as burdens.[3] And whilst caring for a person with dementia (PwD) can often feel like a roller-coaster ride, getting care right in dementia is something to be immensely proud of, both for the individual and to demonstrate a civilised caring society.

Carers (i.e. people in regular caring roles) have been traditionally defined as either formal or informal. Formal implies a paid, professional carer in the home, community or a nursing home setting. Informal means unpaid care, usually provided by a family member or friend. Care itself can vary widely from 'keeping an eye out' and being vigilant to a need for help, to support with 'instrumental activities' such as paying bills, transport to an appointment or help with medication, to more intensive support with 'basic activities of daily living' such as dressing, eating and personal care and hygiene. Whilst formal and informal care are often thought of as either/or, the reality is that, for many people in receipt of care, it is a mixture of both. Even for people resident in a nursing home receiving formal daily support, the family will often augment with some form of input. The important thing in this situation is for formal and informal carers to work together and avoid conflict, as this creates an impossible situation for the person in the middle. Unfortunately, the popular media craves stories of formal carers acting improperly, which eclipse the reality of most care being of a good standard.

Care in dementia

Is care in dementia different? What care do PwD need? Although it may be assumed that the care need trajectory for PwD is simple to quantify and predictable, the reality is different. Even with a relatively simple physical impairment, such as a broken leg, meeting care needs may be complex. It will be a function of not only the impairment, but also the personality of the person being cared for, their preference for their care and the way it is delivered, as well as the personality of the person delivering the care. Do they deliver care in an assertive way, or do they react to need? Do they enjoy the carer role and is this evident in the care they deliver? Even if carer and 'caree' are aligned, the calibration of care takes time. And this is even more true in dementia where the brokering of care arrangements can be very complicated.

Understanding the mercurial needs of a PwD is challenging, and the carer's ability and experience in meeting these needs can vary considerably.

There is a relative lack of information regarding how best to respond to care needs in dementia. Most would assume there is a linear and predictable increase in care requirements that moves from a light touch of care involving welfare checks, perhaps some cleaning and assistance from family in paying bills, towards assistance with cooking meals and showering, moving into more intensive support in an institutional setting, and help with personal care and feeding. This might also mean initially being supported (informally) in the home by a spouse, children or friends (their roles and jobs permitting) starting in an ad hoc manner, perhaps initiated by a crisis or specific issue, and then in a more regular metered manner in anticipation of a need. There may be a point where it is decided, collaboratively or more paternalistically, in response to family concerns regarding coping at home, that a move to a nursing home is made. Here it is assumed that the loved older one will live in a safe and supported environment until the end of their days. But, this 'average' or presumed care trajectory is not representative.

In reality, pathways into and through care vary. It must be remembered that people are individuals, not just in health, but also in illness, and that disability is as varied as ability. This makes the delivery of person-centred care a challenge.

Dichotomies of care can exist on many axes: paternalistic versus autonomous care; proactive versus reactive care; transactional care versus social support. Ideally care should be didactic: both flexible and responsive to care needs and dependencies, whilst simultaneously maximising autonomy and independence. Dementia throws a spanner in the works in achieving this, as there is usually a mercurial progression of the illness. Some days will be characterised by improved lucidity where paternalistic and authoritarian delivery of care will be inappropriate, and a perceived threat to autonomy. Equally, other days will be marked by more confusion, necessitating a more proactive and directive approach to maximise comfort and dignity. Some carers have an innate talent to flexibly respond to these challenges. Others will need support and supervision to achieve this. Irrespective of carer experience, the relationship between carer and the PwD is the foundation of effective care. And, as we will discuss later, there are many challenges to the formation and maintenance of these caring relationships.

Carer 'typologies' (profiles)

Mary will ask later what kind of carer you are and what kind of carer do you wish to be? To answer these questions, it is helpful to look at the some of the typologies of carers that we find in care settings. The intention here is not to be pejorative or criticise people's intuitive caring styles, but rather to use these caricatures as the foundation for further examination of how to be the carer you want or need to be. And although these carer types are discussed as carer traits, the reality is that every carer would have entered all of these states at one time of another, prompted by the situation at hand.

Broadly speaking, there is a spectrum of carer engagement, ability and aptitude, and that has been described theoretically, but both Mary and I have also witnessed the spectrum directly in memory clinics and care settings. And although these carer typologies are generally applied to informal or unpaid carers, my experience is that they can describe types of formal carer as well.

One research team, Brown et al, describe a continuum of carer involvement that ranges from no involvement, through being an informant, to being a collaborator in care and then becoming an expert director of care.[4] They also describe a situation of the family carer being a 'co-client', where the focus of any intervention will be on the carer as well as the patient. This has relevance for later discussion about how best to support carers in their role. The carer continuum could also be extended further to include a carer who either consciously, or unconsciously, sabotages attempts by others to care, for a number of potential reasons which will be examined later. However, at the other end of the carer spectrum is the expert carer, who is a fully engaged co-ordinator of care.

The expert carer

As mentioned in earlier chapters, Mary and I have often encountered extraordinary examples of expert carer family members providing excellent nuanced and person-centred care. Sometimes, when I encounter these experts, I feel that I and the medical model have little to offer. The expert carer seems to have intuitively grasped the dialectical nature of good care that simultaneously addresses instrumental or basic care needs, and yet also maximises autonomy and rehabilitation potential. The expert carer is able to respond to the mercurial challenges of a PwD, stepping up on difficult, more confused days, and taking a more background role on better days where self-governance is easier. The expert carer is also aware of his/her own limitations and of working as part of a care and health system, which is often imperfect and bureaucratic; he/she demonstrates resilience and perseverance in brokering arrangements with care providers when additional paid formal care is needed. Expert carers understand the competing demands of care, and that autonomy and paternalism are competing concerns, and that different situations demand a greater focus on one or the other. Similarly, they never lose sight of the person being cared for and recognise the importance of social input as well as instrumental and more intensive support.

Expert carers also understand the personal demands of the carer role and set realistic expectations of their own performance, having a healthy perspective when things invariably do go wrong from time to time. They also understand that dementia can present management dilemmas, particularly when approaching end of life, and that the discordance of opinion that often occurs is a healthy reflection of the complexity of these dilemmas.

Lastly, expert carers realise that they are people, not robots, and that caring for a PwD on a regular basis will provoke strong feelings in the carer. The expert carer realises that these cannot be avoided, but can be reflected on, rather than being acted on automatically in a lightning rod manner, transmitting additional difficulty in an already emotionally charged situation.

The carer in difficulty

What sits at the opposite end of the carer spectrum? Before describing the characteristics of this type of carer, I want to reiterate that in caricaturing this type, the intention is not to embarrass or criticise the inadequate carer, rather to use this extreme description to demonstrate pitfalls that all carers will encounter at some point. This will then form a prelude to a discussion of how carers can help themselves to remain able and robust in these difficult roles.

As well as the occasional joy of encountering an expert carer, Mary and I also encounter 'the carer in difficulty'. This type overlaps with the 'stressed carer', 'the depressed carer', 'the angry carer' and the 'begrudging carer'. All merit some description and again it is important to highlight that even the expert carer has been one of these types at one time or another. Accordingly, it may be better to conceptualise these as carer states rather than types per se. That aside, the clearest early indication that I have encountered a carer in difficulty is, in my view, the 'chair swivel test'.

Usually in my memory clinic, my chair is pointed in the direction of the 'patient', with the occasional swivel towards a carer or relative when they are talking. However, I try to keep my body and face positioned towards the patient for most of the time during a consultation. At times, however, I realise that my chair has been swivelled towards the carer for most of the consultation and it dawns on me that the carer is the true patient, or the person in most need during the consultation. Typically, the PwD is calm and accepting of his/her impairment and all the distress and difficulty is located in another – the family carer.

At first glance, there is disproportionate reaction from the carer to the situation. For example, a person with an early diagnosis of dementia may have an objectively mild cognitive impairment (with a near normal cognitive test), and not be experiencing any non-cognitive problems, such as depression or anxiety, be functionally independent, not requiring any formal care support and with no currently identified risks. He/she may, however, be less fastidious with dressing or make-up, becoming less proficient at managing finances, or becoming less active at home, content to stay in the house and disengage with previous activities that he/she did regularly.

There have been times in the memory clinic when discussing such a scenario, when a carer in such a situation suddenly 'decompensates' – that is, he or she expresses anger, frustration, anxiety, fear or depression and cannot be reassured in the moment. At this point, my chair has been swivelled towards the carer for most of the consultation, and there is an explicit realisation that this is a 'carer in difficulty', or that the carer is more a 'patient' than the PwD. But why is this the case? The reality is there can be many reasons.

Caring for a loved one with dementia is a challenging task and it is unlikely that anyone placed in the role can become an immediate expert in such a complex position. And as with any difficult vocation, experience and knowledge are needed in equal measure to navigate a nebulous array of complex challenges. For example, encouraging a family matriarch to accept help when her hygiene starts to decline; deciding whether it is best to re-orientate or validate when a PwD becomes disorientated; discussing with a nursing home manager a concern regarding the way one carer communicates with a loved one; deciding whether it is best to prioritise autonomy over risk; or what is the minimum frequency of showering when there is care refusal. Some will find all of this too much. These situations provoke a number of emotional reactions, often linked to feelings of inadequacy that for many will be intolerable.

Thoughts on sustainable care in dementia

More is being written about care in dementia, and there are now a number of trials of different carer support packages to determine what is most effective in supporting carers in their carer roles to deliver effective and person-centred care. Rather than provide here a narrative review of these trials, which have been well summarised by others,[9] I thought I would share my own personal thoughts on being a carer, from both a professional and personal perspective.

- Look after yourself first. This advice is the same as that given during a flight safety demonstration. Apply your own oxygen mask before helping others. A depressed carer can't give their best. The martyr carer is unavailable when they fall in a heap after being an on-call carer 168 hours per week for a year. An anxious carer with insomnia is rarely fully present when they are exhausted all the time. The point here is that carers need to feel rested, fed and ready to face the day ahead before they can take on any responsibility. Respite, in some form or another, be it several hours on a Thursday morning or two weeks each summer, is not an optional extra for carers in a long-term carer role. Paid carers also need professional support and supervision.

- Create a realistic 'vision of care'. This vision can act as a guiding principle and as a fair contract between all people concerned. Good care is 'best fit' care, not 'perfect' care, as this is about as common as unicorns. Good carers do their best, in the context of available resources. They work with, not against, professionals and have realistic time frames when it comes to brokering paid care arrangements. They do not self-flagellate when something goes wrong, as this is the nature of the beast with dementia. Similarly, they work proactively with health and social care professionals to avoid difficulties and risk, using pragmatic and proportionate strategies.

- Investigate the core principles of acceptance and commitment therapy (ACT). This cognitive behavioural approach promotes good mental health through a commitment to values-based living and an acceptance of the diversity of experience, both good and bad.[10] Carers could benefit from this approach through a commitment to value-based care (usually person-centred), and an acceptance of the implicit difficulties in the carer role. On a more practical level, ACT can help support carers through difficulties in the care process by enabling them to accept their own emotional reactions to the often difficult present situation, retaining a commitment to their own values and that of the person needing care, and taking a pragmatic course of action, available to them in the current context, to best satisfy all the considerations present.

- Lastly, I believe that the traditional distinction between paid and unpaid, formal and informal carers should be challenged. I think that informal carers should access the same educational programmes and support that paid carers can access. Similarly, I think paid carers would benefit from contact with family members and informal carers outside of the actual care environment, so that perspectives of care from both groups could be explored and reconciled and that carer partnerships could be strengthened.

The consequences of not caring

My last thoughts on care that I want to express relate to the consequences of not caring, both as an individual and on a societal level. Although caring for a PwD brings many challenges, it also brings many rewards. Traditional narratives of care have always focused on the negatives, such as the carer burden, but there is emerging work on the consequences of *not* caring. I think it is useful to highlight these, as this may help validate those in carer positions and further raise the profile and importance of care delivery.

- For all the talk and discussion of carer burden, there is some evidence that caring for others can in fact be good for one's health. In a study by Brown et al, results suggested that providing at least two hours of care each day to a spouse decreased mortality for the caregiver, suggesting that the caregiver's health may actually benefit from providing care.[5]

- When caring and non-caring children of a parent needing care are compared, it is more likely that non-caregivers experience depression than caregivers.[6] This again, conflicts with the prevalent notion that being a carer is inevitably a burden.

- Other research suggests that if a caregiver is experiencing burden or stress, this is less related to the care recipient and more to family dynamics and conflict within the caregiver's family.[7] I can certainly attest to the latter from personal experience.

- Increasing globalisation, technology and care-giving over distance ('astronaut families') may change the future landscape of care.[8]

- The consequences of not caring on a societal level are perhaps more profound, but will not be discussed here, apart from saying that I would suggest that dementia care may be the best surrogate of how civilised and forward thinking a society is. The countries that deliver the best care for those with dementia, in my mind, are those that are best at caring for their older, more vulnerable populations in general. We consider this further in Chapter 8 (page 161).

II. (MARY)

What type of carer are you? Which do you want to be?

What makes someone a carer? The term is used both in a professional sense – of hospital, residential and care agency workers – and in an informal sense referring to spouses, partners, children – even neighbours and friends who, due to circumstances, are the chief support of someone who needs care with everyday living. In the case of dementia there is an essential need. People with dementia cannot manage without support and help. Society has a two-edged (or two-faced) response to care. On the one hand carers are 'angels' who give kindness, compassion, companionship, practical help and support to those in need of their services. On the other, carers are those at the bottom of the heap – people who only undertake this job because they cannot aspire to anything 'higher'.

The difficulty that society as a whole has in reconciling these two roles is the reason why caring as a profession is not valued. There is a further anomaly. Someone who undertakes the role for pay – the professional carer – has a generally low status, receives low pay and frequently has poor working conditions and is exploited by the employer. Someone who is 'thrown' into the role – whose relative or friend develops dementia and who becomes the chief supporter of that person – becomes touched with an aura of self-sacrifice, of shining goodness, almost of sainthood. These people do not undertake the lowly role because they must, or because they are incapable of aspiring to something higher. No! They are to be revered as well as pitied, to be supported and offered help. They are seen as victims of circumstance, almost venerated.

It is not that our society offers enough in the way of help and support even to these perceived saintly victims of circumstance. The role of carer never goes away – people do not cease to need care during holidays or at weekends or even at night. Truly, the carer never sleeps. Society pays lip service to this fact whilst withholding the help and support which might make the role supportable, tolerable – might even make the role enjoyable and satisfying.

The job of the 'informal carer' has a further downside. People with dementia frequently show their worst side to those who are closest to them. The help offered by husbands, wives, partners, daughters, sons is rejected and reviled, whilst the care offered by the agency carer or the healthcare worker in hospital is accepted and appreciated. Thus, the family carer is subjected not only to the stress of the constant alertness required in the caring duties but, at worst, is criticised, suffers aggression, is bullied and intimidated. At best, his/her help is accepted grudgingly and thanks are withheld. It is not easy to work out why this should be but it certainly is so.

Time after time families tell me how upset they are – not so much by the fact of dementia, since sooner or later most come to realise that the PwD is truly unable to help themselves – but by what they see as the ill-logic, the ingratitude, the failure to give loving responses in return for loving help freely given. It is possible to rationalise this behaviour as due to the emotional certainty that the PwD has, that they can do what they like and help will not be withdrawn; the 'you always hurt the one you love' syndrome. It is also possible to understand with a logical mind that PwD no longer understand cause and effect and that they react emotionally and unthinkingly in the manner of a child. It is even possible to see that someone may feel humiliated when help is given with personal care by a loved one, but not by similar help given by a professional.

Such rationalisations are of only limited help. Family carers *are* emotionally involved with the one they care for, and rejection of help, displays of anger and aggression, and failure to show appreciation are hurtful. When I am training professional carers, we spend quite a bit of time working on the maxim that they should 'not take it personally' but this is not an easy thing to convey to family carers who have years of previous relationship experiences – good or bad or both – to colour their interactions with the PwD.

Why use the term 'carer'?

Is there a problem perhaps connected with the very word 'carer'? A spontaneous discussion during a social event involving both PwD and carers raised this question. One newly diagnosed person raised the topic. He objected to the term 'carer', claiming that it made him feel patronised. He felt that he did not need a 'carer', but only someone to offer him a little help occasionally. His spouse agreed. She found the term demeaning which echoes the suggestion of the low status accorded to carers by society. She also objected to the change in attitude of people with whom she interacted when she explained that she was now a 'carer'. A lively discussion followed, and at some point the question was asked, 'What other term could be used?' It became clear that the people present who had had a diagnosis of dementia almost all disliked the term. They suggested a better descriptive word would be 'helper' or 'supporter'.

No consensus was reached by the carers who were present, but many said that they saw no need for a collective term. Most of them would prefer to be known as the spouse, son, daughter or friend of the one they were supporting. When this subject was raised with a group of professional carers, the resulting discussion and conclusion reached were quite different. They did not want to be called helpers or supporters or friends, or even the new, frequently-used term, 'care-givers'. As one of them declared to me: 'We are happy to be called carers because we care.'

How can you make proactive rather than reactive caring choices?

Professional carers choose to be such, but most family carers would say that they had the role of 'carer' thrust upon them rather than it being a matter of choice. Since dementia usually comes on rather slowly it might be more correct to suggest that carers 'drift' into the role. Many of the decisions that carers have to make are made under less than ideal conditions. The PwD is found to be less able to manage the activities of daily living so the carer begins to assist. Perhaps on one occasion the PwD gets lost when out, or becomes confused in a non-routine situation. The carer reacts (they go searching, call the police, alert the neighbours) and the current situation is dealt with.

It is common for carers to assume that an event like getting lost is a 'one off' situation, but even so they may take steps to prevent its reoccurrence. However, such behaviour is reactive in nature. Because dementia symptoms are 'person specific', it is not possible to say exactly how someone's condition will deteriorate, or what minor or major 'crisis' the carer might have to deal with. Experienced health professionals, such as community psychiatric nurses and dementia support workers and advisors, are able to explain possible scenarios and steps to take in anticipation of these events.

Informal family carers usually find it hard to think ahead and plan, partly because they have a natural inclination to ignore unpleasant future possibilities, and would prefer to believe that 'their' cared-for person is unlikely to progress through any of the more unpleasant or disturbing behaviours. But acceptance of the progress of dementia, and anticipation of future problems, can bring empowerment. It used to be quite difficult to persuade people to give power of attorney for financial affairs. People used to tell me that they would 'do that when it was needed', but the widespread dissemination of information about LPAs has resulted in many people drawing these up earlier in life, with the result that life is simpler for both them, and those who care for them when the time comes that they are no longer able to manage their financial affairs. If people were to think ahead about other matters and make similar arrangements, the result would be major empowerment and a smoother caring path.

How can we make person-centred care meaningful?

Person-centred care is a 'buzz phrase' that is used in most literature about caring, and in almost all training material. What does it mean? The phrase was coined at a time when caring tended to be 'task orientated'. Carers in care homes were supposed to deal with the tasks of washing, dressing, toileting or feeding those they cared for and caring was seen as the process of carrying out these tasks. 'Person-centred care' was supposed to mean that carers should see, and get to know, the people they cared for as people with a past history, with likes and dislikes, tastes and emotions, not just as a 'dementia case'.

Amongst family carers the concept of person-centred care is inherent. The person for whom they are caring is known to them – has been known to them in the past as a *person* and the fact that they have dementia is overlaid on that person. They are and always will be 'dad who has always been a miserable person' or 'mum who always liked helping others' or the spouse with all the past joint history of a life together, including making a home and bringing up a family, caring for pets, making joint friends, sharing holidays and hobbies and enjoying good times and enduring difficulties and hardships, and offering and accepting solace and comfort. So, in this sense there is a dramatic difference in the caring given by a family member and the caring given by a professional paid carer. Family carers don't really need to learn about 'person-centred care' because they are already giving it.

Professional carers working for a care agency or in a care home, or as live-in carer to someone with dementia, may not have the background information to allow them to really give 'person-centred care'. Most care agencies and care homes ask families to complete a history and personal preference statement when they begin to offer care, and this is considered to be good practice. The problem arises when this information is not communicated to the hands-on carers by their management. I visit many care homes and in most the carers tell me that that they have not read a history, or even been briefed by senior management about those they are expected to care for.

The reasons for this are varied. Most often the notes are locked away 'in the office'. Occasionally the resident may have a 'personal folder' which is displayed in their room, perhaps containing photographs, a life history, a description of likes and dislikes, together with a copy of the care plan and perhaps a list of regular medication. The daily carer seldom has time to peruse this document in any depth. Some carers do not have the skills in written English to understand the history. Some home managers feel that the appropriate place for this document is in the manager's office, where they assure me that 'the carers can ask to look at it at any time'. Seldom is the history of the resident easily accessible to the daily carer so that they can check an item quickly. This lack will be discussed further in Chapter 8 (page 172).

Care agencies working in the community are often guilty of the same lack of communication. The person who does the initial assessment is usually a senior 'care manager', and they will take a history and complete a care plan which should be agreed with the family of the person being cared for and – supposedly – with the PwD. Daily carers will then be scheduled to visit and carry out care – sometimes quite intimate personal care – often without any in-depth briefing of the past history or the likes and dislikes of the person they wash, dress and help in the toilet. Over time, regular carers both in the residential home and in the community, do learn about the people they care for. Good carers take a pride in getting to know and befriending those they look after. But a proper briefing and a good introduction at the start would ease the way and might help prevent an abiding resentment at being 'looked after' on the part of the PwD.

How to avoid being bullied by the condition

In other books I have discussed the situation where the PwD – and who thus is no longer fully in control of his or her logical thinking – can become the family 'bully', ruling the household and making unreasonable demands on those around them. In this chapter we are looking instead at the situation where the carer and family become bullied *by the condition*.

In many cases the diagnosis of dementia is regarded as so catastrophic, so overwhelming, that the family allow their entire lives to revolve around it. Every action, every routine and every event in life is subject to the dementia. Normal routines are no longer adhered to, and attitudes change completely. The family – in particular, the main carer – find themselves so governed by the illness that they no longer feel as if they are normal members of society. In some ways, the present emphasis on educating the general public to understand dementia encourages this attitude unintentionally. It is as if the PwD and the family around them are no longer 'normal' members of society. Whilst the intention of this emphasis on educating the public is well meaning, intending as it does to encourage a better understanding of the effects of dementia, it may be that the constant talk of 'dementia-friendly high streets' and 'dementia awareness', along with terms like 'dementia friends', encourages society to set PwD apart and to believe that they need special treatment and special environments.

This of course is not the intention behind these well-meaning ventures and initiatives. What PwD – and their carers – want is to carry on living in the manner to which they are accustomed with their interests and pastimes catered for, their friends', neighbours' and families' continued interaction, and society's acceptance of them as before. However, the diagnosis bestows upon them a change more significant than a diagnosis of diabetes or heart disease. Suddenly they are set apart as 'special' and 'different', requiring a change in attitude by their friends and neighbours, different facilities such as day centres and care agencies, and cautious approaches by anyone who comes in contact with them.

Of course, a better understanding and more considerate attitude on the part of social communities is not wrong. Special facilities and 'dementia-friendly communities' are all positive steps in allowing PwD to function within the community. But given that the mean age of the population is rising, there is a clear indication that there will be many more PwD living amongst us, and wanting and needing to function within the society in which they reside. Rather than thinking about 'dementia-friendly communities', society might want to look at a general simplification of ways and means so that this functioning is facilitated for everyone, and 'special facilities' and 'dementia-friendly initiatives' are no longer a particular requirement. Once we have considered how we want our dementia to be (see Chapter 1, page 1), we might like to think about how we want to be accepted by those around us once we too are affected by dementia.

REFERENCES

1. Martin LG, Preston SH. *Demography of Aging*. National Academies Press, 1994.

2. *The Economist*. The demographic time-bomb. *The Economist* 2008; Aug 27.

3. Koerner SS, Kenyon DB, Shirai Y. Caregiving for elder relatives: Which caregivers experience personal benefits/gains? *Archives of Gerontology and Geriatrics* 2009; 48(2): 238-45.

4. Brown J, Nolan M, Davies S. Who's the expert? Redefining lay and professional relationships. In: Nolan M, Davies S, Grant G (eds) *Working with older people and their families*. Milton Keynes: Open University Press; 2001: 19-32.

5. Brown SL, Smith DM, Schulz R, et al. Caregiving Behavior Is Associated With Decreased Mortality Risk. *Psychological Science* 2009; 20(4): 488-94.

6. Amirkhanyan AA, Wolf DA. Caregiver stress and noncaregiver stress: Exploring the pathways of psychiatric morbidity. *The Gerontologist* 2003; 43(6): 817-27.

7. Scharlach A, Li W, Dalvi TB. Family conflict as a mediator of caregiver strain. *Family Relations* 2006; 55(5): 625-35.

8. Baldassar L. Mobilities and communication technologies: Transforming care in family life. In: Kilkey M, Palenga-Möllenbeck E (eds) *Family Life in an Age of Migration and Mobility: Global Perspectives Through the Life Course*. London: Palgrave Macmillan UK; 2016: 19-42.

9. Cooper C, Mukadam N, Katona C, Lyketsos CG, Ames D, Rabins P, Engedal K, De Mendonça Lima C, Blazer D, Teri L. Systematic review of the effectiveness of non-pharmacological interventions to improve quality of life of people with dementia. *International Psychogeriatrics* 2012; 24: 856-870.

10. Twohig MP. Acceptance and commitment therapy. *Cognitive and Behavioral Practice* 2012; 4: 499-507.

Chapter 7

Improving the emotional experience of dementia

Summary

- People with dementia may experience different 'realities' but all individual realities are subjective.

- The most important question is whether people with dementia are happy within their own cognitive 'reality'.

- The principles and practice of mindfulness may help both the person with dementia and their carers.

- Orientation and validation are both helpful approaches in dementia and can be flexibly applied to the situation.

- Emotional fluency and awareness are generally maintained in dementia, and carers need to have insight into the effect of negative emotions on the person with dementia.

I. (MARY)

Living an emotional life – is dementia a threat or an opportunity?

Can there be any benefits in a diagnosis of dementia? Most people would give a resounding 'No!' to this question, given that the general impression is of a devastating disease which affects the ability to live everyday life independently, is known to be progressive and puts a high burden on near family and carers. It is true that dementia causes those people affected to become more dependent on others, to become depressed and frequently to become more anxious and confused. The lives of family and friends of people with dementia (PwD) can also be adversely affected and, indeed, the diagnosis of dementia can cause a great deal of stress, distress, anger and despair to the close family of the person who is diagnosed. It can seem absurd to even contemplate any suggestions of a beneficial effect.

Most people know that dementia affects the brain and that this causes the people affected sometimes to behave differently from how they used to, and to react in a manner which now seems wrong and abnormal. There is a general belief in society that PwD frequently behave aggressively and even violently towards others and this raises a general feeling of trepidation and even fear in those who have little experience of, or association with, someone who is cognitively challenged.

The allocation of denial and acceptance roles

People who have dementia generally need more support than others and they may be unable to function independently or to live alone. They may need help with everyday activities, such as washing, dressing and simple household tasks. They may be unable to manage their own finances or to complete application forms, to answer the telephone or to make their own appointments and social arrangements. In fact, a complaint often made by medical professionals is that PwD are most often defined by what they are *unable* to do. At the memory clinic and other medical appointments, the carers will often launch into a litany of failures and faults and what seems like a stream of complaint about progressive loss of ability. It can seem strange to hear husbands, wives, and close family members recite a history of aberrant behaviour and failure to reach acceptable standards, to clinicians and support workers.

The reason why carers generally relate these facts is because they are afraid that the clinician will not take their referral seriously. Many believe that the clinician will be 'taken in' by the ability of the person awaiting diagnosis to appear to behave in a socially adept manner, as though they have no cognitive problems. Generally speaking, carers will not begin the consultation by relating the things that the person awaiting diagnosis can still do ably and well. People who have cognitive problems, on the other hand, often express their conviction that there is nothing wrong with them. If they do admit to any 'memory problems', they are likely to assign these to natural ageing and to make light of, or to find (frequently plausible) excuses for, any disability. This is common and reflects the recognised internal struggle between the acceptance and denial of deficits in a PwD. These reactions can then be projected into the family with individuals occupying denial and acceptance roles.

We have a difference apparent here in the way that PwD and those closest to them view their cognitive disabilities. Individuals can then become locked into their various perspectives of the current situation and the future. Persons with a diagnosis often assert at routine follow-up memory appointments that they are 'fine', that their memory problems have become no worse, that they are not depressed or worried in any way (although occasionally people will express some concern about their carer), and if asked about the future they will often not seem to comprehend the question. Carers on the other hand will usually point up a deterioration in cognition and in the ability to carry out activities of daily living, they may assert that the PwD seems depressed or anxious, and the carer frequently expresses concern about the future. This is a vivid illustration of the way that dementia affects the brain and thinking patterns not only of the individual PwD, but also of the carer–patient 'dyad' (two-person unit, see p.144) and family systems.

Logic and emotions

When someone has dementia the part of their brain which is controlled by the hippocampus is compromised. This is the part of the brain that deals with logic, systems and reasoned argument. It is the area of the brain which is constantly worked on and developed as we grow by our parents, and those around us who have a part to play in our development and maturity. As parents and teachers and others involved in helping infants grow and mature, this is the part of the brain that we constantly appeal to. Think of statements like these:

'You need to go to bed because you have to be fresh for school tomorrow.'

'You can't have a sweet now because it is teatime soon.'

'If you share your toy with your brother he will share his with you.'

We do not use these tactics with babies. Why not? It seems obvious. We don't appeal to a baby's reason because their brain is not developed enough for this to work. Imagine how stupid it would seem if we appealed to a newborn baby in the following terms:

'Please don't cry. Mummy needs her sleep to be fresh for tomorrow.'

'Don't fill your nappy now – we are about to go out.'

'You must go to sleep so your brain will develop properly.'

Let us look again at what is happening to someone who has dementia. We are not talking now about physiology – how the neurons deteriorate or how the brain atrophies. Let us give consideration to the effect that the dementia has on the way someone thinks and reacts. We could say that the part of their brain that deals with reason and logical thought is deteriorating. The PwD cannot control this deterioration. Bit by bit, day by day, they become less able to follow an explanation, to conduct a sequence of actions, to understand a set of instructions.

This fact is remarkably difficult for most people to understand and come to terms with. The tendency is for carers to treat the PwD like a child with learning difficulties – to simplify their conversation, to repeat instructions loudly and clearly, to distract them from difficult situations, and to exchange meaningful grimaces and subtle glances with the other 'normal' people around them. Up to a point, this strategy succeeds. It is sensible to speak more clearly and slowly to someone whose thinking processes are slower than usual; it may reduce stress levels in a PwD if we distract them from difficult scenarios; and it may make carers feel more in command of the situation if they can signal to others that they are acting in a certain manner to cater for the needs of the PwD.

However, there is more to the brain than logical thinking and reasoning. The human mind also has 'feelings' – emotional reactions – to what is happening around the person. Many books have been written and motivational courses designed in order to attempt to teach people to 'control' their emotions. Usually, it is suggested that we control our emotions by using our logical and reasoning abilities – the equivalent perhaps of giving ourselves 'a good talking to'. Sometimes, instead, it is suggested that we control one emotion by using another. For example, if we are feeling sad and depressed we can try playing uplifting music, watching comedy films or taking part in physical exercise and activities which distract us. There are some enlightened writings which acknowledge that emotions can be positively engaged, but by far the bulk of our upbringing, training and teaching in life is dedicated to teaching us to overcome our emotional side and encourage our logical reasoning abilities.

When the brain is affected by dementia, logical thinking and reasoning ability are affected quite early on. However, the amygdala – the part of the brain that is the integrative centre for emotions, emotional behaviour, and motivation – is less affected. People with dementia who have trouble processing logic and reasoning do not have a similar problem with their ability to feel emotion. Indeed, as far as research can show, PwD still feel happy, sad, afraid and so on, even after they can no longer speak or recognise people they know well, even when they need total support to live their lives. It seems, though, that most people – including many well-meaning carers – are unable to adjust their own behaviour and thinking to accommodate the continuance of emotional experience, along with the decrease in reasoning ability of the person they care for.

If someone has a broken leg we do not assume that they could walk on it 'if they tried'. We do not suggest that they listen very carefully whilst we explain how to walk. We do not try to divert their attention so that they can walk without thinking. No. Instead we set the broken bone and maintain it in position with support (a leg-plaster). We allow them to rest the leg. We give them a crutch to aid movement and we accept that walking will be slow and difficult until the leg is healed. Similarly, if someone has part of their brain which is not functioning we should make allowances. We should try to keep the parts of the brain that do function in as good order as possible – by encouraging social interaction, physical exercise and general health. We should allow the brain to 'rest' when it needs to by not demanding actions which are no longer essential. We should supply a 'crutch' using memory aids, providing unobtrusive help and support. We accept that everything cannot be as it once was because this brain is not what it once was.

It is important, though, that society should recognise the relative importance of the emotions which come to predominate when logical thought and thought processing are deteriorating. Society in general does not much like domination by the emotions. 'Civilised' people should learn to control emotion and apply logic and reason to manage their everyday life, it is thought. But what if we can no longer use our logic and reasoning to help us come to terms with emotions? Suppose we are unable to understand and work out why we feel sad or happy? Imagine if we feel these emotions overwhelmingly, but we are unable to deal with them by a change of scene, by talking through our feelings, by taking actions to alleviate the misery or express the happiness. Imagine being no longer able to speak coherently enough to tell anyone how frightened you feel or how angry. What might you do? How might you try to express yourself? Perhaps you would try to hide somewhere, or to run away and escape. Or you might shout and get angry. Perhaps if no one made any effort to understand, you might try to use physical methods to show them how you feel.

Applying logic to a mind governed by emotion

Most people are well meaning. Carers will often try to understand.

Generally, though, what people try to do is to apply their logic and reasoning to the emotional turmoil of the PwD. 'What is wrong, dear? No, you need to go through this door. There you are. Now let's find you a seat. No, don't go back out. You need to sit down quietly. Sit here. Margery! Come and sit down. We'll get you a cup of tea. Why do you want to go out? There is nothing out there. You have only just come in.'

When it comes to caring for PwD, perhaps sometimes women may have an advantage over men. As I've said, dementia tends to affect the hippocampus first (the part of the brain which governs factual thinking, logic and reason). People with dementia find it more difficult to follow a reasoned argument or a logical line of thought. However, the amygdala (the part of the brain which, as I have said, governs feelings and emotional memories) is much less affected to begin with. This means that increasingly PwD are using their 'emotional' responses to make sense of the world around them. Someone who cannot remember who a person is may still know how they 'feel' about them – for example, if the person makes them feel happy and gives them a sense of security. Similarly, if their ability to use logic and reason to interpret a situation is damaged, then a PwD may work on what a situation 'feels like' rather than what it actually is.

Traditionally, men have been seen as more logical and likely to use reason and to try to 'solve' a problem, whereas women have been seen as more likely to empathise and to try to understand how someone else feels about a situation.[1] It is regarded as natural for a man to try to apply a reasoned approach – many women will be familiar with this, and many men will be in despair at the response to this approach from a woman: 'You just don't understand!' It is equally natural for women in general to empathise and understand the feelings of the person they are speaking to.

So women who are carers of PwD may be better able to

empathise and to 'go with the flow' of the feelings of the person they care for. The behaviour of PwD can sometimes seem strange – even bizarre – but if we get behind the behaviour and understand that their communication is based on feelings, not facts, often things make much more sense. Carers need to get away from logic and reason and look at what someone may be feeling on an emotional level. In my experience, some women carers may find this easier to do. This in no way implies that women are better carers than men, simply that they may find it easier to cope with the change from logical to emotional expressions of thought.

There is another analogy with childhood and infancy which is frequently avoided by professionals when dealing with dementia. Sensible parents do not allow children to rule the household and do whatever takes their fancy. This is because children do not have the maturity and ability to reason and to understand the consequences of their actions. It may be a controversial statement, but the simple fact is that neither do people with advanced dementia have the ability to reason and understand the consequences of their actions. The demented person who becomes aggressive and hits their carer is certainly not to be blamed because they are unable to follow the reason as to why they should not do this. Their action is instinctive, like that of a child who throws a tantrum when stopped from doing something that is not allowed. However, the sensible parent does not allow the child to have his way because of a tantrum. By a variety of methods, the demanding, unreasoning child is taught to realise that he will not get his own way if it is not appropriate.

Caring for a PwD is not the same as caring for a growing child, of course – although sometimes carers say that it seems like it. The brain of the child is maturing and is making new connections every day. What the child does not understand one day, he or she may begin to understand on a day in the near future. The brain of a PwD is losing connections every day. What was understood one day may be lost the next. What is evident is that the ability to feel emotions is not as quickly lost – and may never be lost at all.

The 'right' feelings

Suppose we turn our attitude to PwD completely upside down. Let us suppose – just for a moment – that PwD, those who feel rather than reason, are in a better place than those of us who are able to reason and use our logical abilities. Let us suppose that they are right, right to feel afraid, right to feel unhappy, right to feel angry and frustrated. There are things they could once do that now they cannot, things they want to do that they are prevented from doing, places they want to go and other people stop them from going there. Some PwD are not angry. They seem placid and compliant. They tell you that they do not worry (to which the carer inevitably replies, 'No, I do the worrying'), and that they are content and mostly happy. If we continue our supposition for a while we can see that they are right to be happy and complacent. They no longer have worries or anxieties. Someone else manages their day-to-day problems and sees to their needs. When we look at things from this vantage point we can accept that the emotional way of thinking is a valid way. We might then ask ourselves why society sees dementia as something wrong.

We as a society need to accept our emotional state and self and give recognition to the many benefits of living emotionally. When we acknowledge and give credence to the emotional thinking of a PwD we instinctively know how to help them best. We also cease to expect them to conform to our 'normal' way of thinking and reasoning, recognising and accepting the emotions of dementia and tuning in to them as a valid part of life. In this way relationships may find a new dimension rather than being seen as a 'loss of the person/past companion'. How does this work? Someone who has dementia sees things emotionally rather than logically or rationally. If they feel unhappy they will demonstrate this without inhibition. If they feel frightened they will express this.

Once we realise this, it is possible to accept the freedom it gives. When interacting with PwD we no longer have to 'second guess' them. We do not have to try to 'see beyond' the face value as might happen when interacting with other people. There is no need to use our intuition or to try to get behind what someone is saying. Generally, PwD say how they feel or show it by their body language. There is a wonderful lack of subtlety and subterfuge. Problems arise when we do not take these feelings at face value. We are so used to dealing with people who disguise their feelings, who show a 'public face' to the world, who do not say what they mean and who do not mean what they say.

When we try to work out why a PwD is saying what they are saying or doing what they are doing, we are on the wrong track. Yet so many learning texts and training packages for carers are specifically aimed at doing just this. Suppose instead, society were to rethink the attitude that PwD are mostly 'thinking in the wrong way' and to accept that this different way of using the attributes of the brain is as valid as the logical and reasoning way that we have become accustomed to?

Getting in touch with emotions – our own and those of the one we care for

A great many books have been written on the theme of 'managing our lives better by controlling our emotions'. A common suggestion is that 'we cannot control the behaviour of others but we can control how we think and react', and theories about how to manage our emotions and how not to allow them to affect our behaviour and our reactions abound. With all the conditioning of early childhood and the pressure to remain 'in control', it can be very difficult to understand that there is any benefit to living emotionally. The PwD has no choice in the matter. Their emotions are paramount and their fears, joys, love, likes and dislikes are a vital part of their life.

When I am training professional carers I like to ask them what their reaction is to someone in their care who says that they want to go home. As mentioned in Chapter 5 (page 99), most carers tell me that they assume the person is slipping back in their memory and looking for a place that they used to know as home. They suggest that the best tactic is to distract the PwD or talk about their long-lost home. A few recognise that fear may be behind the expressed wish, and that the desire to 'go home' is an expression of a wish to be somewhere safe and familiar. When these carers understand that fear is behind the expressed wish, they can change their behaviour towards the person who is afraid and try to comfort and reassure rather than distract.

The times when PwD exhibit their emotions are the times that allow carers to get in touch with their own emotions. If someone is unhappy we can try to identify with that, and help them to become happier. If someone is cross and frustrated because they cannot do something which previously they found easy to do, then it is time to acknowledge that anger and frustration and perhaps identify our own anger and frustration at the situation as well. Once the understanding and acknowledgement are in place then we can act to find a solution – perhaps making an adjustment to a routine, or adding in a mechanical aid to help future actions. It is most important first to acknowledge the emotion, and only then to use our logical mind to find a solution.

II. (NOEL)

The different cognitive realities in dementia

There is curiously little research about how PwD experience time. A common belief would be that people with advanced dementia are living in the past, fuelled by observations of autobiographical inaccuracies and confusing the past and present. Alzheimer, for example, noted Auguste Deter to be confused about whether her mother was alive or dead and took this to mean she was 'living in the past'. The most dramatic examples of this, which Mary and I encounter, and which can be very difficult for surrounding family, is when the death of a child has been 'forgotten' and there is repeated questioning about their whereabouts. However, I do not interpret these experiences as supporting the idea of 'living in the past'. Rather, a person with advanced dementia is living in a universal now, or a temporal reality, which is a conflation of past, present and future. Without the usual faculty of episodic memory, which anchors our experiences on a linear timeline, a PwD can be living in a temporal reality without the usual subjective expectation of what there is to come and what has been.

A neuro-anatomical explanation of temporal disorientation in dementia focuses on selective atrophy and malfunction of the hippocampus – a snail-shaped structure buried deep in the brain which has an important role in memory as well as logical thought. However, we know that such a complex and layered experience of memory and time cannot be localised, or reduced to one part of the brain. I do not think that medicine, even in 2017, can provide a clear explanation of how and why time is experienced differently in dementia, and whether this experience is necessarily abnormal. I would rather turn to a group of Buddhists and physicists to ask whether the PwD's experience of time is pathological or normal, useless or enlightened.

I often think that art, rather than science, may be able to

answer, or at least pose, this question more helpfully, or in a way that may be reassuring to the PwD, rather than the empty explanation of hippocampal or brain dysfunction. The experience of watching Samuel Beckett's play *Waiting for Godot*, for example, crystallises the complexities (and absurdity) of existence, and that there is no one true objective reality for all. I think that most people would agree with this point, but because dementia remains doggedly viewed as a *pathology of the brain* rather than an *experience of the mind*, people often do not allow themselves the freedom to explore different cognitive realities in illness, and in particular, whether these realities are as valid as the reality of people who are *well*.

It seems perverse that as a society we are very happy to accept that each night most of us involuntarily participate in bizarre, non-linear and surrealistic experiences in the form of our dreams, and that we often find truths and meanings within this experience, and yet we instantly dismiss the different cognitive realities of PwD as being due to brain dysfunction and inherently having no reality. I am not suggesting that *Waiting for Godot* should necessarily be included on every dementia carer's curriculum, but it would form a useful discussion prompt about whether the existential realities within this play mirror those of PwD, and have meaning or value. Are the characters existing in a kind of timeless reality without any clear forward (or backward) narrative? Does this create experiences that are meaningful, or do Vladimir and Estragon (the play's protagonists) simply react to the current situation in an absurd and thoughtless way? I suspect Samuel Beckett would answer yes to all questions.

Probably the most important question here is whether PwD are happy within their own cognitive realities. I think the answer to this question is complex, because our emotional state fluctuates according to our perception of reality. But I think the main difficulty for PwD is that their new cognitive reality is imposed by dementia, rather than being a state entered on a voluntary basis.

I have come to believe, through observations, particularly in the nursing home, that the cognitive experience for PwD ranges from the euphoric to the nightmarish. This may relate to the individual's pre-morbid tolerance for altered conscious states, and how wedded he or she was to a clear linear, cause-and-effect narrative through their lifespan. It may also relate to the inherent ability of the individual to view themselves and their thought patterns non-judgmentally. However, although the cognitive reality may be very different for every person who is cognitively impaired, I believe that most are happy within their new cognitive realities.

There is interesting and important research that has examined the relationship between memory and happiness, specifically that they are largely independent variables.[2] I often make an explicit point to people in my memory clinic, that *you do not need a perfect memory to enjoy life*. I tell people that the key to happiness is to enjoy the moment, rather than dwelling on the past or the future, and this advice is the same for people with or without a memory difficulty. It is, of course, not reasonable to expect that every moment will be happy, as anxiety and distress are a normal part of life, but if we allow it, these emotional states pass like clouds in the sky.

Living in the now – mindful dementia

This naturally brings us on to a discussion of mindfulness. I often say in my memory clinic that my advice to PwD is the same as to people without. That is, to try to live life day by day, and not get too caught up in worrying about the future or ruminating about the past. Really notice what is happening in the now and embrace that, rather than being distracted by what you may think is around the corner. Life is lived in the now, not yesterday or tomorrow. I also ask carers to consider whether their life (and anxieties about their loved one) could be improved by living by these principles. Very often I find PwD and carers in my memory clinic have already intuitively adopted a 'take it day by day' strategy and this group tends to be more content and less daunted by the future. This approach to *living life in the now* is in keeping with the principles of 'mindfulness' or 'mindful living'. It borrows heavily from Buddhist ideology and the practice of meditation, and has become an increasingly popular approach to depression, anxiety and other forms of mental distress.

Mindfulness aims to educate about the inherent human tendency to judge experiences, and how the mind often wants to change an experience in order to avoid distress or anxiety. Practising mindfulness also illuminates how attached we become to how things *should* be, and the fantasy that things can always stay the same. A diagnosis of dementia will inevitably be viewed as a threat to our concept of self and the world, but the reality of life is that we are constantly challenged by multiple insecurities and perceived threats. If we can somehow learn to embrace, or at least accept, the insecurities inherent in a human lifespan, then when a diagnosis of dementia occurs, the ability to live fully in the now will not be as threatened.

Over the course of my memory work, I have often wondered whether PwD are inherently more mindful, or at least positioned by their illness to live mindfully. For those with more pronounced episodic or short-term memory loss, they will necessarily be compelled to live in the now, or at least the conflation of before–now–later described above. This may be largely a passive experience imposed by their dementia. Mindfulness, however, as per Buddhist philosophy, implies an active practice, usually through meditation, in order to train the 'attention muscle' of the mind to be present fully and non-judgementally within a moment, even if the current moment is full of worry, pain or a distressing mood.

As I have said, people with dementia who have severe impairments of episodic memory have no choice in the matter, in that a new temporal reality is imposed, timeless, mindful or otherwise. Bishop et al, in a 2004 psychology consensus statement on mindfulness, state that mindfulness is:

> ... closer to a state than a trait because ... its evocation and maintenance is dependent on the regulation of attention while cultivating an open orientation to experience. As long as attention is purposely brought to experience in the manner described, mindfulness will be maintained, and when attention is no longer regulated in this manner, mindfulness will cease.[3]

Given that attentional deficits are a common component of cognitive impairments in dementia, this could be interpreted to mean that dementia and mindfulness are incompatible. However, both Mary and I believe that much can be done to improve the experience of daily life with dementia, for both the PwD and the carer, and that mindfulness may be very useful here.

What is mindfulness?

I think I need to describe mindfulness in more detail before discussing strategies to help towards this aim. Mindfulness has been classically defined as a skill to ease personal suffering, by paying attention to the experience of the current moment, and is usually developed by the Buddhist practice of meditation. A more contemporary psychological definition of mindfulness, provided by Bishop et al (2004) is:

> ... an approach for increasing awareness and responding skilfully to mental processes that contribute to emotional

distress and maladaptive behaviour.[3]

They go onto to say that:

> ...in a state of mindfulness, thoughts and feelings are observed as events in the mind, without over-identifying with them and without reacting to them in an automatic, habitual pattern of reactivity. This dispassionate state of self-observation is thought to introduce a 'space' between one's perception and response. Thus mindfulness is thought to enable one to respond to situations more reflectively (as opposed to reflexively).[3]

For PwD and their carers, mindfulness may be of particular help in dealing with automatic and catastrophic thoughts regarding the impact of dementia on their future lives, by realising that feelings of panic and grief triggered by the diagnosis may be temporary events in the mind that can be observed rather than elaborated on. Even if the PwD is not able to practise mindfulness personally, it can have indirect benefits if practised by the carer, because of the preservation of emotional recognition in dementia. As discussed earlier, the carer–patient bond can be strong enough that they can be considered as a 'dyad' (two-part unit), rather than two individuals. And if one half of that dyad can be self-soothing, through mindfulness or any other practice, then this often results in reduced stress in the other.

What are the principal techniques used to become more mindful? Bishop et al believe that mindfulness is composed of two broad processes.[3] The first is the ability to focus attention on the current experience, creating a medium in which to become more aware of the volume of mental events triggered by a present situation. The second involves developing a non-judgemental stance to these mental events 'that is characterised by curiosity, openness, and acceptance'. It is not the intention of this book to provide a comprehensive guide to mindful meditation, particularly when there are many existing resources. Readers may wish to refer to early texts of Kabat-Zin, who was responsible for the modern revival of mindfulness in the 1980s,[4] or refer to resources from the Oxford Mindfulness Centre,[5] which is an internationally recognised centre of excellence for mindful practice. I think anything which educates people about the flexibility of mental processes is helpful.

Mindfulness may be particularly helpful for carers in dementia, not just because of its role in stress reduction, but because it educates the carer about the inherent subjective nature of mental processes, and in particular, how there is no 'correct' or superior cognitive experience in any given moment. This may then help reduce the unhelpful or automatic imposition of the cognitive reality of the carer on to the PwD. This will now be described in more detail, looking at other therapeutic approaches that include validation and mindfulness.

To correct or not correct? Orientation versus validation approaches in dementia

A common post-diagnostic question in the memory clinic from carers is *how* to approach disorientation or cognitive misunderstandings. Typical scenarios include when a PwD becomes disorientated in their own home and asks when they are returning home. We have spent some time above discussing subjective realities in a more abstract form, and whether the imposition of one reality onto another is always correct or justified. However, when posed this question by carers, Mary and I recognise the need for practical advice as well as illustrative theory. I think the dilemma of how to respond to disorientation and distress is a good example of how dementia care often involves a discussion of both the abstract and the pragmatic.

This particular problem has attracted considerable research interest, perhaps because it is so common, and is split into two camps – re-orientation (or reality orientation) or validation. Mary and I usually preface the conversation by saying that these two approaches are not mutually exclusive.

- **Reality orientation** is probably the most commonly used approach for disorientation and distress in dementia and involves reminding the PwD of forgotten facts about themselves or the environment, either verbally or using visual memory aids.[6] Although the approach is intuitive, there is concern that frequent reality orientation can constantly remind PwD of their memory deficit and deterioration, rather than reassure.

- **Validation:** As a response to this, an alternative approach of 'validation' was developed by Naomi Feil, which advocated the validation of feelings in the moment, rather than focusing on confusion.[7] Validation therapy recognises that a PwD may retreat into the past as an active attempt to avoid feelings of being lost and alone, and, that by validating this experience, rather than reorientating to factual reality, conflict and stress between carer and PwD can be avoided.[8] Critics of this approach warn that by becoming too focused on the emotional content of confusion, simple explanations for this, such as pain, hunger and thirst can be easily overlooked.[2]

Whilst reorientation and validation approaches are presented as opposites, the reality is that both can be helpful. Mary and I take time to explain this, and that whilst one approach may work on one day, another may be appropriate the next, and that carers should use their gut instinct about which to employ in a given situation. We also caution that they should not be too hard on themselves if things do not go to plan. We also discuss how distraction can be a useful tool in addition to reorientation and validation, when responding to disorientation and distress.

To illustrate these three approaches, we return to the previous example of a PwD becoming disorientated in the home and asking to go back home. To say, 'Don't worry, we're already at home' would be a response based on reality orientation, whilst a response of 'Why do you need to go home? Is there anything I can do?' would be more validating. Saying 'We'll go home in a little while' could be considered as being based more on distraction, whilst taking the PwD outside for a five-minute walk, returning back home and announcing, 'Here we are', is arguably a combination of all three. Rather than present these three approaches as evidence-based strategies that must be employed with precision, we emphasise how creativity and flexibility can be used, not just to reduce distress in the PwD, but also to help the carer with what he/she is feeling; and to encourage a reflective, rather than reflexive, approach to situations, consistent with principles of mindfulness.

We also emphasise that there may be no need to respond, if disorientation occurs without distress or difficulty, going back to the initial point about whether the imposition of one cognitive reality onto another is always justified or helpful.

Different emotional realities in dementia

We have spent some time discussing the different cognitive realities that occur in dementia and how existing psychological approaches, such as mindfulness and validation, may help us understand ourselves and improve the experience of dementia. It is equally important to explicitly discuss emotional realities in dementia and how existing psychotherapies offer some wisdom around improving emotional experience in the condition. The first point to reiterate is that, unlike cognition, there is no linear decline in emotional abilities. Whilst there can be significant emotional dysregulation in some dementia syndromes, such as emotional disinhibition in frontotemporal dementia (FTD) and easy lability (extreme variability in mood) in vascular dementia, emotional fluency and awareness are thought to be remarkably preserved in Alzheimer's disease. This does make it more difficult to describe a panacea to address emotional conflict for all these clinical situations; however, the broad principles described below can be helpful for all PwD and their carers.[9]

Avoid emotional paternalism

Given that emotional fluency and awareness are generally maintained in most PwD, it is important that carers avoid an 'emotional paternalism' that can arise from the assumption that the emotions decline in parallel with cognition in dementia. This leads to a position of assumed emotional orientation in a given situation or conflict. All parents would have experienced fall-out from a similar assumption of emotional superiority in an argument with their children. The reality of emotional appraisals is that they are by their very nature subjective, and there can be no 'true' emotional response to most situations. As emotions are such automatic aspects of daily human experience, we rarely give thought to their subjectivity, or how accurately we appraise them in others. To be aware of both these aspects is the first critical step in reducing the impact of negative emotions both in life and in dementia.

Investigate talking therapies

Different theories exist to explain emotional expression in humans. These can be helpful in understanding those who are frequently affected by distressing emotional states and have a lack of control over their feelings. Most people with psychiatric conditions such as depression, anxiety, eating or personality disorders can benefit from a psychological approach to their symptoms. People with dementia and their carers are no different, although this has only become an interest in research relatively recently. Many different schools of psychotherapy exist, from Freudian psychoanalysis through cognitive and behavioural therapy (and variations thereof), to counselling. Although these models of talking therapy appear very different, they share a common premise that emotional states are not automatic reflexes to a given situation.

Like mindfulness, other psychotherapies aim to educate the client or patient that their emotional reactions to given events and circumstances are buffered by other processes, such as unconscious defences (psychoanalysis), particular thinking styles (cognitive therapy), behaviours (behavioural therapy) or thinking in isolation (counselling). The rationale is that by examining other processes that occur in the mind, the experience of emotions can be changed. Cognitive behavioural therapy (CBT), for example, aims to help feelings of low mood by examining the relationship between feelings, thoughts and behaviours, and emphasising that thinking and behavioural patterns that maintain depression can be changed.

Most recent research into the use of talking therapies, like CBT, in dementia has focused on the carer. Although this can be initially thought to bypass the PwD, there can be real benefit to both carer and PwD. Any approach that strengthens the mental resilience of the carer in the carer–patient dyad (two-person unit), will benefit the PwD. This is the rationale behind 'systemic therapy' sessions for child and family, typically used to help a child with emotional distress. Because the child's distress exists in the family 'system', there are often changes that can occur in the system that will benefit the child. This approach avoids apportioning blame for a child's distress, instead looking creatively at a child's social circumstances, and the family's reaction to a child's emotional response, to see what can modified to improve matters.

A similar approach can be used in dementia with emotional

distress. Here, emotional responses (such as anger and worry) can be viewed as emotional behaviours which then provide a framework to modulate either the behaviour itself, or the distress caused to the PwD or carer. At its simplest level, any emotional response can be investigated to look for patterns of both 'precipitants' (triggers) and consequences. This behavioural analysis can reveal previously unseen triggers or reinforcing actions that maintain a particular emotion.

Although behavioural approaches can be criticised for being a simplistic view of the complexity of human feeling, Mary and I have witnessed at first hand how adopting a different approach to feelings can be empowering to carers and PwD. It is beyond the scope of this book to provide a comprehensive summary of CBT or other psychological approaches in dementia; we urge you to seek out the many existing excellent guides to using these techniques, including Naomi Feil's guide to validation therapy listed below.[8]

REFERENCES

1. Levine S. Sex differences in the brain. *Scientific American* 1966; 214(4): 84-90.

2. Banerjee S, Smith SC, Lamping DL, Harwood RH, Foley B, Smith P, et al. Quality of life in dementia: more than just cognition. An analysis of associations with quality of life in dementia. *Journal of Neurology, Neurosurgery & Psychiatry* 2006; 77(2): 146-8.

3. Bishop SR, Lau M, Shapiro S, et al. Mindfulness: A proposed operational definition. *Clinical psychology: Science and practice* 2004; 11(3): 230-41.

4. Kabat-Zinn J, Hanh TN. *Full Catastrophe Living: Using the Wisdom of Your Body and Mind to Face Stress, Pain, and Illness.* London: Piatkus; 2013.

5. Oxford Mindfulness Centre. http://oxfordmindfulness.org

(accessed 23 July 2017).

6. Douglas S, James I, Ballard C. Non-pharmacological interventions in dementia. *Advances in Psychiatric Treatment* 2004; 10(3): 171-77.

7. Feil N. *The Validation Breakthrough: Simple Techniques for Communicating with People with 'Alzheimer's-type dementia'*. Health Professions Press; 1993.

8. Feil N. Validation therapy with late-onset dementia populations. *Caregiving in dementia: Research and applications* 2014: 199-218.

9. Rankin K, Baldwin E, Pace-Savitsky C, et al. Self-awareness and personality change in dementia. *Journal of Neurology, Neurosurgery & Psychiatry* 2005; 76(5): 632-39.

Chapter 8

The politics of dementia and the nursing home

Summary

- Ageing is not a purely biological process and the experience of ageing is influenced by political, economic and social structures. Dementia is no different.

- The source of most distress for people with dementia and their families in the UK is increasing difficulties in brokering care and support.

- Activism around better dementia care has been curiously absent. What appears to be lacking in public debate are conversations about care and care reform.

- The commodification of disease, including dementia, in healthcare systems has had consequences.

- The lives of people with dementia are most affected by crises in care, rather than by finding a cure.

- Many dividing practices operate in dementia. Dividing practices describe any practice where people are objectified and then divided from others.

- Life writing by people with dementia (PwD) is a good starting point for more meaningful dementia activism. This is because it shifts the debate away from the search for a cure to the experience of people living with dementia.

I. (NOEL)
The political economy of dementia

This chapter, focusing on the politics of dementia, aims to provide some context to dementia in 2017 and, in a similar vein to previous chapters, to argue that it is not the absence of a curative magic bullet that creates the most distress for the person with dementia (PwD) and their families, but the way that people with the condition are treated by health and social care systems and greater society. The corollary of this is that, in the absence of a 'cure', if social and political systems could respond to dementia in different ways, then much of the distress caused by dementia could be mitigated. This chapter should really be entitled 'the political economy of dementia', an adaptation of 'the political economy of ageing', a phrase which was coined in the early 1980s aiming to describe how ageing is not just a biological process, but is modulated by political, economic and social structures.

The concept of the political economy of ageing has generated research into the effects of economics, capitalism, social policy and class on the ageing process,[1] and by implication, focused attention on how social policy and politics need to change to redress many of the socioeconomic inequalities that develop as people age.[2] If this chapter can provoke the reader to consider the broader influences on the social experience of dementia, away from the narrow biomedical perspective, then it has achieved its purpose. If the reader is also politicised by many of the injustices experienced by PwD, perpetuated by existing structures and processes, then this is also a welcome effect!

The story so far – a history of dementia activism

In Chapter 2, the history of 'dementia' as a pathological entity over 700 years was examined in brief. As a diagnostic concept, dementia continues to evolve. Similarly, the way that dementia has been treated by health and social policy makers has also changed over time, and whilst some countries, such as Japan, Germany and Denmark, are rising to the challenges of an ageing population and the increasing numbers of PwD by implementing significant structural reform, other countries' responses have been less positive or relatively muted. Keeping the concept of the political economy of dementia in mind, it can also be seen how broader policy and economic shifts have had significant and often damaging effects on PwD. I remain perplexed by how little debate there is regarding the political economy of dementia, which remains eclipsed by the brighter fantasy narrative of the search for the miracle cure. Particularly in Europe, where there are significant regional differences in policy responses to population ageing and dementia, political aspects of dementia rarely receive public attention.

In the UK, although the rhetoric of the 'economic time-bomb of the ageing population', and fears of exponential increases in dementia prevalence frequently enter the headlines,[3] this has not translated into a real policy shift, such as social care reform. Maintaining the status quo has long been the favoured government policy response to the threat of increasing morbidity (poor health) in the older population. An example was the Department of Health (DoH) dementia strategy, launched in 2009, which had laudable aims to improve the awareness, diagnosis and care experience of dementia through 17 key objectives. However, the strategy was launched without any funding and has not been successfully implemented due to financial constraints.[4] GP scepticism regarding the benefits of early diagnosis,[5] questionable evidence regarding the available interventions,[6] lack of resources in primary care[7] and resistance by the public to the intrusiveness of the biomedical model[8] also limited its effect.

In my view, the source of most distress for PwD and their families in the UK is the increasing difficulty in brokering care from a social care system which has suffered from repeated disinvestment and separation from health. The latter was an early '80s Thatcherite attempt to inject free-market efficiencies into public health and social care systems. This has resulted in a legacy of split health and social care and 'dividing practices' that specifically disenfranchise older PwD. These remain under the radar of public consciousness until any of us is personally forced to navigate this divide, usually in a crisis situation.

This is not to say that dementia never enters public and political debate. Perhaps the last time that it evoked significant activism was 15 years ago, at the time that the National Institute for Health and Social Care Excellence (NICE) decided that donepezil, the first cognitive enhancer and sole drug licensed for use in dementia, should be reserved for people with moderate Alzheimer's disease. By implication, this meant that people with newly diagnosed and milder forms of the disease, as defined by a mini-mental state examination (MMSE) score, needed to wait until their disease progressed before being prescribed the drug. This health policy also mandated that as people's Alzheimer's disease progressed from moderate to severe, donepezil, which was expensive at the time, be stopped, even if the person had benefited from the drug previously.

Although cognitive enhancers are moderately effective at best, this event was significant in the history of dementia activism in the UK for several reasons. First, it highlighted the healthcare rationing practices that operate in medicine. Second, it also raised questions about the artificial division of PwD into three severity categories based on a single MMSE score that determined access to treatment. However, perhaps the most intense 'donepezil activism' was fuelled by the idea that dementia sufferers were being denied a 'cure'. Unfortunately, there has been little notable dementia care activism since the donepezil and NICE controversy.

Since the expiry of the UK dementia strategy in 2015, which purported to be a 'diagnosis-to-death' strategy, policy responses to dementia have been focused on increasing 'formal' diagnosis rates. The DoH argues that dementia diagnoses remain too low in the UK,[9] compared with expected prevalence figures, despite other evidence that suggests that these estimates may in fact be too high.[10] Prevalence of dementia can also vary dramatically when different diagnostic criteria are used.[11] The rationale for increasing diagnosis rates is that support for the PwD can only begin after diagnosis. But diagnosis, particularly in the very early stages, is difficult. Early diagnosis is prone to error, particularly in environments like a hospital where cognitive examination is confounded by a multitude of other factors which may influence how the person responds to tests.[12]

Furthermore, formal diagnosis targets ignore the fact that dementia is often diagnosed informally within the family or in healthcare, and that the clumsy application of a premature 'formal' dementia diagnosis can cause real harm and distress to people. This is especially true when older patients are screened inappropriately for cognitive impairment in the context of a delirium, or acute physical illness in hospital, and then automatically referred to a memory clinic without knowledge or consent. Or a situation may occur where a family member's dementia has been reframed by the family as 'forgetfulness' or as 'memory glitches' in order to reduce fear around a dementia diagnosis. The benefit of the imposition of a formal diagnosis in this context, when the patient is safe, happy and supported by informal networks, can be rightfully questioned.

In my view, the best referrals that I received in the memory clinic were those made by GPs who knew, assessed and counselled their patients well, so by the time of their appointment with me, if a diagnosis of dementia was made, there had been a helpful preamble to my discussion. Most direct referrals from the hospital, where cognitive screening had been financially incentivised, were lacking in any personal history, usually based on a solitary MMSE test score (often carried out when the patient was physically unwell), and without any discussion with the patient or their family. Other concerns that incentivising earlier diagnosis can undermine the doctor–patient relationship have been raised.[13] Diverting resources away from already poorly funded post-diagnostic support may be another unintended consequence of the drive for earlier and earlier diagnosis.

Consequences of commodifying disease and dementia

Since the post-Thatcher split of provider and purchaser in the health sector, there has been an increasing market-driven focus on the commissioning and provision of health and social care. For example, in the planned introduction of 'payment by results' (PBR) in mental care. Anderson (2009) explains that PBR is:

> … a fixed tariff payment system … that reimburses acute care hospitals for the type and number of patients treated … and by linking provider income to activity, the tariff is expected to provide incentives for higher output and lower costs per patient.[13a]

This increasingly market-based context of health care delivery and the 'commodification of disease', including dementia, has potentially negative consequences. It is feared that the introduction of a PBR system will increase heath inequities within the health economy.[13a] This is because it is already suspected that negotiated tariffs for the care of older PwD are too low, meaning that health care providers will not be fully remunerated, and therefore resourced adequately, to manage PwD properly. This may also lead to treatment for PwD being effectively disincentivised, as providers prioritise the treatment of simpler conditions in younger patients.

This commodification of disease therefore disadvantages older patients, particularly with complex conditions like dementia or significant medical 'co-morbidities' (other health problems). Existing targets and financial penalties within the NHS already work against the needs of older people with cognitive impairment and confusion, an example being the previously mentioned four-hour rule in accident and emergency, meaning that older patients routinely change ward settings at least three times in three days, worsening any pre-existing disorientation and confusion.[14]

A care crisis rather the cure crisis

Many excellent voluntary sector charities exist, such as the Alzheimer's Society, and work hard to raise the profile of dementia research. Whilst any strategy that encourages public and professional discourse on dementia is always welcomed, the focus typically remains on the biological aspects of the condition; namely, diagnosis, treatment and research for a potential cure. What appears to be lacking in public debate are conversations about care and care reform. Headlines regarding 'the epidemic of Alzheimer's disease' need to shift away from the absence of a cure towards the absence of clearer future policy around care.

There is a care crisis, not a cure crisis. And the former can only be addressed through reform of social care funding. Currently in the UK, healthcare is free at the point of delivery. Social care, by contrast, is means-tested. This means that the majority of PwD and their families will have to fund their own care, which is now delivered by the private sector.

The popular media loves horror stories about sub-standard care in failing nursing homes, or narratives about abandoned relatives living at home. What is rarely discussed are the inherent difficulties that most people face trying to broker and fund care packages and residential home placements in an increasingly complex provider landscape, with less and less guidance from local authorities. It is very rare that the installation of some formal care input is not a stressful event for PwD and their families. This stress is magnified by financial worries. Intensive home support, or a placement in a nursing home, can easily cost £1000 a week. Few families have sufficient liquidity to immediately pay for this, and the selling of a family home in order to pay for such care adds another layer of emotions. People are often shocked that social care is means-tested and that they will have to fund their own care until their assets and savings fall below a threshold for state assistance.

It is beyond the scope of this book to decide what is the fairest funding solution to meet the needs of the majority of PwD and their families. Nor is it the remit of this book to endorse any one specific plan for funding adult social care. Fortunately, in the UK, there have already been several comprehensive reviews of this question, with the Wanless and Dilnot reports being the most recent examples. The *Wanless Social Care Review* was published in 2006 and considered a number of potential responses to the care-funding dilemma. For example, a universal system with free personal care to all; or a partnership model of funding; or a limited liability model where care would be means-tested initially, and then be free after several years.[15]

Wanless's concluding recommendation was that a partnership between the individual and the state was the best and fairest model to deliver a minimum standard of care. Wanless et al suggested that state funding of two-thirds of the overall cost of a care package would be fair, and that additional private contributions could be matched by the state. However, as this model would have increased social care costs by about 50 per cent, his recommendation was not implemented.

A more recent high-level review of care funding, by a commission led by Dilnot in 2011, also made a number of specific recommendations regarding care funding, essentially based on Wanless's third option of limited liability for care costs.[16] Dilnot suggested a £72,000 cap on the total contribution that any individual would be expected to contribute to their care. However, the general living costs in a residential care home, of around £7000 to £10,000 annually, would not be included in this.

To put these funding proposals in some kind of international perspective, it is important to note that other countries' responses to the question of care funding have varied widely, from the lack of any funded state response in developing countries, where care remains almost exclusively a family responsibility, to more comprehensive and universal models of funding seen in some Scandinavian countries, such as Denmark. Other countries have adopted more novel solutions, such as the social care insurance model in Germany, where people pay additional ring-fenced taxation to fund future care, and Japan, which has decided that all people above the age of 65 should never have to pay more than £500 per month on care. Japan also has an ingenious older volunteer scheme, whereby older people who volunteer in care receive credits for their own care if that were ever to be needed. A more idiosyncratic response has come from Singapore, which criminalises children who neglect their parents' needs!

The many dividing practices in dementia

Before looking at reasons why there is little dementia activism at present, and what an ideal advocacy platform might look like, I want to discuss the principle of 'dividing practices'. Again, the specific intention is not to politicise you, the reader, but rather to expose the many boundaries that PwD routinely face in health and social care. As well as creating obstacles, any of these dividing practices represent an opportunity to query existing systems and act for change.

The term 'dividing practice' was originally coined by Foucault, a French philosopher, to describe any practice where people are objectified and then divided from others, or aspects of the self are divided.[17]

What dividing practices operate in dementia care? We have already discussed some of the differences between health and social care in the UK, particularly how the former is (currently) a free universal system, whilst the latter is means-tested (in England and Wales but not Scotland). And how care packages that address social needs are means-tested whilst health-related interventions are free. This distinction creates a dividing practice that complicates routine dementia care. Unless a PwD's condition has deteriorated to an extent to meet 'continuing *health* care' funding, their needs will be considered social and any care package will be subject to means-testing.

But this division of needs as 'health' or 'social' is often quite an arbitrary and perverse practice. Personal hygiene, assistance with nutrition and hydration as well as mobilising (moving about), are all generally regarded (or divided) as social needs rather than health needs, despite all of them being fundamental to good health. Social isolation has toxic effects on health,[18] yet is regarded as a social problem. And yet care around these needs, such as care packages or regular social input, are subject to means-testing and 'brokerage' in the private care system.

Conversely, if a PwD's care is coordinated by a member of a Community Mental *Health* Team, assistance with attending a social support group, or going to an Alzheimer's café, will be free, as this is provided by health, not social, care. The reality is that health and social needs in dementia (and in general) are inextricably linked, and this false dichotomy of health and social needs maintained by the false division of health and social care systems creates enormous complications. Although there are frequent attempts to reintegrate health and social care in the UK, the reality is that two systems have been so structurally divorced over the last 30 years, any real reconciliation is unlikely.

Earlier in this chapter, we discussed how the practice of dividing PwD into several groups of severity based on MMSE score led to rationing of treatment with cognitive enhancers when they were first introduced. Dividing practices are an intrinsic aspect of medicine. People are diagnosed, or divided, into 'well' or 'not well'; dementia or not dementia. These divisions can have both positive and negative implications, not just in terms of prognosis but also in terms of access to medication or other forms of help and support.

Take the distinction drawn between mild cognitive impairment (MCI) and early dementia. Often it is very difficult to make this distinction with certainty. And whilst the prognosis of MCI is better, with between one- and two-thirds remaining stable and not progressing to dementia, a 'diagnosis' of MCI compared with early dementia has some negative implications. As funding for memory clinics and dementia services remains suboptimal, it has been necessary for many health and third-sector services and commissioners to set specific criteria for subsequent support. This means that a person with a diagnosis of MCI, who may need exactly the same information and support as a person with an early dementia, will be denied these. Similarly, a person with early dementia may be offered a trial of donepezil, whilst a person with MCI may not be offered this.

Another example of division is dementia aetiology (cause) or subtype. A person with vascular dementia may be denied the option for a cognitive enhancer trial in contrast to a person with Alzheimer's disease, despite some evidence of similar effects being seen in vascular dementia.[19] The boundary between normal ageing and dementia also becomes increasingly blurred as we enter late life, and the point at which someone with advanced age is deemed to require care is often socially determined.[20]

One of the most potent dividing practices that operates in dementia care is when people are divided into risky and non-risky groups. If a PwD is labelled as 'risky' and 'lacking in capacity', then this will usually mobilise a response to mitigate risk, even at the expense of personhood and liberty. The ethics of this are beyond the scope of this book, but it is noted that the exponential rise in applications for deprivation of liberty (so-called DoL safeguards) for PwD in nursing homes is fortunately starting to garner more public attention.[21]

Why has care activism been so absent?

We have discussed throughout the book that the predominant view of Alzheimer's disease remains to think of it as a brain disease that requires a cure, rather than as a condition that is increasing as a consequence of an ageing population, hence necessitating structural changes in how we plan and resource care as a society. This has meant that existing activism has been largely focused on increasing funding for research for a cure, rather than reforming care. Chaufan et al (2012) argue that while the medicalisation of senility and Alzheimer's disease has aroused interest in the problems of ageing, such as dementia, it has also undermined advocacy for care reform. They argue that in an:

... environment of fiscal restraint and small-govern-

ment ideology, policy approaches promising a 'cure'
were likely to prevail over those of 'care' as it feeds
the hope ... [that] effective treatments or a cure for AD
will derail the 'explosive' future costs of caring.[22]

It really seems that dementia has the worst of two worlds.
Whilst most dementia activism focuses on the biological aspects
and the need for research funding into a cure, care needs are
regarded as a 'social problem' which receives little public
advocacy or attention. Although there are parallel advocacy
platforms regarding ageism, loneliness and other age-related
social issues pursued by third-sector organisations like Age
UK, there is little direct linkage to dementia activism, which
remains more biologically focused. Coordinated 'silver' activism
on multiple fronts, rather than the single-issue activism that
currently exists, may be the way forward.

What would ideal dementia activism look like?

We mentioned in Chapter 5 how PwD might benefit from being
seen as having a disability, rather than a disease. In particular,
we looked at how governments have responded to disability
by changing laws to improve the physical environment and to
make social life more accessible to all citizens. The disability
movement has also been very successful at shifting the focus
away from bodily impairment to discrimination and prejudice as
being the real causes of disability.[23] If a cognitive disability model
was also adopted more widely, then this would encourage more
critical scrutiny of current environments and how they may
disenfranchise people living with cognitive impairment and
dementia. Marks reminds us that if we 'think about the needs
of people with learning difficulties, sensory impairments or
mobility problems, our social environment may well be more

sensibly organised for everyone'.[24]

The main assumed historical obstacle to increased participation in dementia activism has been that the cognitive impairment in dementia has prevented PwD participating.[25] Fortunately, the rise of patient representation in the NHS has started to counter this view, and PwD and their carers now increasingly contribute to dementia service governance and strategy. Participation of this kind is vital to provide real insight into the experiences of people using dementia services, and preventing the phenomenon of 'otherness'. This occurs when policy issues surrounding dementia are seen as the problems of 'others', rather than a problem that belongs to all of us as a connected society. The circulation of dementia narratives, or accounts of experiences of PwD, helps neutralise otherness by publicising the universality of the experience of PwD.

A good recent example is the work of Keith Oliver, a retired headteacher living with dementia, who has taken an active and prominent role as a service user envoy in the NHS, sharing his experiences with health and social care professionals and the public. In his preface to *Welcome to Our World – A Collection of Life Writing by People Living with Dementia* he describes the work as 'not just another book about dementia' but rather one that 'is written by a group of people who each have a diagnosis of dementia, who want to share some stories from their lives alongside expressing some thoughts surrounding inhabiting the world of dementia from the inside'.[26]

I think that this kind of work should be the starting point of any meaningful dementia activism. This is because it helpfully shifts the debate around dementia from scientific cure and discussions of the amyloid burden, to the lived experience of PwD and the daily difficulties or obstacles they may face. This is consistent with the thoughts of Ruth Bartlett, who sees two emerging themes of dementia activism as 'gaining respect' and 'creating connections' with others.[27] Her third mode of dementia activism, centred around protecting the self against decline, is also a recurrent theme in Keith Oliver's work, as there is no doubt that maintaining and improving social connectedness for PwD is a potent way of addressing decline – as recommended in Professor Kitwood's work discussed in Chapter 4.

Visibility is also another starting point for effective dementia activism, which not only counters marginalisation and otherness of PwD, but leads to increased participation in health consumer groups. However, there needs to be some radical change in how people in nursing homes can achieve greater representation and visibility in any advocacy, as the nursing home remains the environment most vulnerable to failings in dementia care policy. As a result, Mary spends the remainder of this chapter focused on the nursing home, examining causes of and potential responses to care failures.

II. (MARY)
The nursing home

The final residence of most PwD is the residential care home or nursing home. Some fortunate few manage to live their last days in the house they have lived in during their family life, or the private home they have moved to in retirement, but, whatever the good intentions of spouse, family or friends, most PwD are consigned to a care home at the end. The reasons for this are varied – challenging behaviour, carer exhaustion and incontinence are most often cited as the 'final straw'.

It is true that most carers set out with the intention of keeping and caring for their loved one at home if at all possible. The high costs of residential care are a major incentive for a start. But we should not ignore the fact that most family carers do understand the benefits to the PwD of spending their final days in a place they are familiar with, and there is a natural reluctance of long-term partners to be separated after years of life together. Nevertheless, it is a fact that very few PwD do not experience, even if only for a short few weeks, the constrictions and the benefits of life in a residential care home. A few, very sociable people, who have perhaps lived alone and experienced the difficulties that entails, actually do better in residential care. These include very nervous and frightened people who dislike living alone if they have been forced by circumstances to do so.

However, my experience is that most of those whom I have supported from the point of diagnosis thoroughly dislike living 'in care' and most of them never become reconciled to it. Carers frequently ask me how they can make mother or father, husband or wife, stop asking to 'go home' – what is the best way to explain to these unhappy people that the place where they now live is 'home'? In truth, you can never hope to do this.

Is residential care necessary?

This book is not the place for a discussion of the benefits or drawbacks of care homes versus 'home' for PwD. There are many circumstances where continued residence in the family home is neither the optimum solution nor even viable. I have personally seen too many carers worn out by their 24-hour caring duties, overstressed, sleep-deprived and exhausted, to suggest that the decision to place someone in a residential setting is arrived at lightly. Indeed, the most commonly recognised emotion felt by those making the decision is that of guilt – guilt at not being able to manage their caring duties, guilt at being separated from their life partner, guilt at not keeping promises rashly made about never 'putting someone in a home'.

In order to understand why residential care becomes necessary we need to consider the true facts about dementia. At first, the PwD can continue to function in his/her everyday life with just a little support. Indeed, there are those with a diagnosis of dementia who continue to live alone for quite some time, although this is never an ideal solution. With regular visits from caring relatives, or from helpers from a care agency, people can be helped to remember to eat, to carry out daily tasks and to maintain a social life. Those already living with a carer – usually a life partner or adult offspring – can function even better. Possibly they may need regular reminders about washing, dressing and appointments, or it may be that the family carer gradually begins to take over chores, such as managing the money, cooking or driving the car.

But dementia is a progressive condition. As time goes by, PwD need more and more support, guidance and supervision in order to carry out everyday tasks. Where initially it was sufficient for the carer to talk them through their ablutions and to lay out their clothes in the order they need them, for example, it gradually becomes necessary for the carer to help them into the shower or bath, to physically wash them and to help them to dress. In time, the PwD loses the ability to initiate activities, so that where they may have been able to help chop vegetables in preparation for a meal or to set the table or to dry the dishes, they may now pick up the vegetable knife and gaze helplessly at the pile of vegetables awaiting attention, or hold the tea towel and wander aimlessly around the kitchen. The carer may find their day consists of a long list of instructions: 'Put your arms out; pull your socks up; come downstairs; fetch the cloth out of the drawer; put the plates on the table; pour your tea; eat your breakfast now; don't get up from the table; finish your food; get your coat on; fasten your shoes; wait on the step for me; get into the car ...' and so on.

This in itself is very tiring for the carer and irritating for the PwD. If we add in the likelihood of the PwD objecting to being told what to do, or initiating an action at the 'wrong' moment (for example walking away across the car park whilst the carer is buying the parking ticket), or wanting to do something which doesn't fit in with the day's planned activity, it can be seen that every day becomes a burden for the carer and a source of constant frustration for the PwD, and this supposes that the carer and the PwD are at least physically fit.

Do you want to live in a care home?

Given that circumstances may frequently make residential care a necessity, it behoves us as a society to look at the quality of life and care obtainable in a community setting and to discuss how often – or how seldom – the highest quality of care is on offer for those we love and care for. One telling factor is that very few of us, before dementia overtakes us, would state that we might choose to end our days in a care home. And yet why is this? Surely for those who are frail, and perhaps disabled, bowed down by the constant cares of maintaining a property and keeping up with even the simple everyday chores involved in daily living, the prospect of being looked after and cared for, of being relieved of the burden of cooking, shopping, laundry, house maintenance and the like, ought to hold some attraction.

People who are able to express their feelings will often quote 'loss of independence' as an objection to moving to a care home, and this is a very real objection. Most homes will describe in their literature the excellent facilities they offer, beautiful gardens, comfortable bedrooms, pleasant communal sitting rooms, perhaps a library or a bar, visiting hairdressers and podiatrist services, convenient medical facilities, a full and varied programme of activities and so on.

Step inside one of these homes and visit the reality. Residents are often chivvied out of their bedrooms and into communal rooms, whether this is their choice or not. Beautiful gardens may be well maintained but are often inaccessible to residents due to locked doors and lack of staff. Less able residents cannot access the library, the hairdresser or the bar without help, which – if they have dementia – they may be unable to ask for. The activities programme is seldom as varied as advertised and scheduled activities are almost all communal so that 'one size fits all'. Above all, residents cannot go outside for a walk, to visit the shops or local amenities unless permitted to by staff. Look closely when you visit. Almost all of these homes have a secure 'entry' code on the *inside* of the door, which prevents residents going out at will.

There are many well-run and comfortable residential homes, and staff are frequently well meaning and caring. In citing the downsides above it is not my intention to denigrate the splendid efforts of many to give a good quality of life to those they care for. What I am pointing out here are the facts, and I am happy to acknowledge the reasons for them. Bedrooms have to be cleaned, for example, and it may be essential for residents to vacate the rooms so that proper cleaning may be carried out. Staff may fear that unpleasant weather, or slippery conditions, may cause residents to fall over and so the doors to gardens may be kept closed, and people wishing to go out are guided away from the gardens.

Shortage of staff may mean that people cannot always be helped to access leisure facilities and frequently they may not even be asked if they wish to do so. Activities are usually managed by a lone 'activity manager' who can only deal with small conformable groups. Leaving front doors open is a security risk with vulnerable people around, and confused people cannot be left to go outside to the local shops or simply to walk the streets in case they get lost. However, taken all together, these facts make understandable the expressions of fear about loss of independence.

It is worth considering what we want from a care home. Many times, carers have said, after relating that their cared-for seems unhappy in residential care and constantly expresses a wish to come home, 'But I must say he is well looked-after! When I visit he is always clean and shaved and properly dressed. I am always offered a cup of tea. His room is neat and tidy.' This type of comment – and there is nothing wrong with the views expressed – perhaps illustrates what carers expect and want from a residential home. I have explained in previous books that what the carer feels is important may differ from what the person being cared for wants. If the family see Mum clean, properly dressed and well fed they can feel satisfied that she is being looked after.

But being clean, properly dressed and having meals presented regularly may be very low on the list of priorities for the person in care. Perhaps what they would like is to feel safe, surrounded by familiar things, and undisturbed. Perhaps they would like to be able to step outside and enjoy the fresh air whenever they feel like it – just as they would at home. Perhaps they would like to go to bed after midnight and stay up watching late-night movies, or to get up with the sunrise and do a spot of gardening before breakfast. Perhaps they desperately miss their husband/ wife/partner and are grieving for their loss. Mostly – because dementia affects the ability to communicate – we have no way of knowing. The truth is that residential care homes are seldom chosen by the person who has to live there, but by their relatives, family and carers. The future resident may often not even see the place where he or she is to live before they are taken to stay there permanently.

Thinking about independence

If independence is the thing most valued – the one criterion which we fear to lose by accepting residential care – are there ways that care homes can foster this feeling whilst still taking care of the practical hygiene and safety issues that families feel are important? There are many residential homes which are licensed for dementia care – yet what does this mean? In my role supporting PwD and their carers I am often asked to advise about the most appropriate homes. I am not allowed to 'recommend' homes, and in any case, even if I did so, it might be that relatives would not agree with my choice. The saddest occasions for me happen when, after relatives have carefully researched, visited and selected the home they think appropriate and been through the heart-wrenching process of settling their cared-for there, with all the attendant emotions of guilt, worry and relief, the home decides that they 'cannot cater for the needs' of the PwD. The relatives then have to go through the whole procedure again and the PwD has to go through a bewildering change, which they are quite unable to understand. Why does this happen? Who is to blame? If the home is registered for dementia care why do they find they are unable to cope with the PwD?

I believe that there is a fundamental failure in the care-home system when it comes to dementia care. Volumes have been written about person-centred care. All the training for carers emphasises this aspect of care – the person is paramount and not the disease. Yet residential care homes are arranged and run according to a 'one size fits all' system, where only lip service is paid to 'person-centred care'. The fact is that dementia is challenging. Those with dementia are confused and unable generally to explain their confusion. They may have lost their ability to carry out many actions of everyday living, but they have not lost their emotional inclinations, their likes and dislikes, their feelings of frustration, anger, humiliation, love, boredom, desire for independence, need for peace and quiet, wish for fresh air, ability to feel pain and so on.

It is true that staff in residential care homes are often involved in an endless 'guessing game' when trying to ascertain the reasons for a certain behaviour on the part of a resident. This is frustrating for both the staff and the resident. Even well-trained staff do not have a supply of endless patience, nor the time to spend in working out the best way to help every individual. Something has to give and usually it is the needs of the PwD. If they express their anger or frustration they are labelled 'difficult' or 'challenging'. The needs of the other residents, or sometimes even the needs of the staff, are accepted as more important than theirs. If concerned relatives protest they are told that they must remove their cared-for to another establishment. The registered dementia home cannot cope with this PwD.

What will it take to change this system?

Changes in expectations

Firstly, family carers must change their expectations. If the paramount requirement is that the person they care for must be clean, properly dressed and fed three meals a day then this is what staff in the residential home will be working towards. No care worker will have time to consider why Mr S is not compliant today if they are under pressure to have the residents in their charge roused, washed and dressed by a certain time. Mr S will have to be roused, washed and dressed whether he wants to be or not because this is the target that the care worker is working towards. If he protests because he doesn't feel well or because he is in pain or perhaps because he just feels like a lie-in, then the care worker's time schedule is disrupted. However much the care worker may understand the needs of Mr S, she is under pressure to achieve her targets and those of her manager and the manager of the establishment. Those needs are dictated by the demands of the relatives of the residents, and by the fixed requirements of bodies such as the Care Quality Commission whose function it is to ensure that care homes achieve a certain standard of care.

Considering the cost

People with dementia need a great deal of attention in order to function well. They need constant reassurance from someone who cares for them in order not to become over-anxious. As the condition progresses they also need assistance with almost every action of everyday living. By the time residential care is considered the PwD will most probably be unable to wash or dress themselves without help, may be unable to use the toilet without help, may forget to eat and drink unless reminded and will almost certainly be unable to prepare a meal or even make a hot drink without help or supervision. They will have ceased to be able to entertain themselves through activities such as reading, playing a musical instrument or carrying out activities such as DIY or craft. When you take all this into consideration, it is no longer surprising that the general conception of a care home is a place where people sit in a circle gazing vacantly into space. It is a great tribute to the dedicated staff in many homes that *any* activity takes place amongst the residents, because all activities require so much carer input.

If we wish life in residential care to be meaningful for PwD then we need to be prepared to pay for a much higher ratio of staffing and a higher quality of staff. What is needed are specially trained, dedicated care workers who can not only ensure that those in their care are clean, properly dressed and fed, but that they are also contented and fulfilled and able to spend their days in activity which is meaningful to them. Care workers of this quality need good training and to be well paid – and there must be enough of them – so that, for example, if Mrs C wishes to go for a walk there will always be someone available to walk with her, or if Mr J wants to try to dress himself, the care-worker assigned to help him has the time to allow him to attempt this. Social interaction is vital for PwD and people can never be replaced by technology in this respect. Society must be prepared to pay for the high standard of care required. Families are frequently taken aback by the high cost of residential dementia care, but they will pay similar amounts for a stay in a first-class hotel on holiday – without the personal care!

Dementia is challenging

I once visited a care home where the manager proudly told me, 'We don't accept anyone with challenging behaviour.' I wondered how this home could claim – as it did – to be a 'specialised dementia care home'. The fact is that PwD are challenging, even if they are compliant and conformable. Quiet, conformable PwD may allow themselves to be helped, may sit where they are told and take their medication without complaint, but they may not be happy or fulfilled. Their very compliance and quietness is likely to imply that they are depressed and that they have 'given up' on life. If you are confused and unable to recognise those around you, puzzled by your surroundings and unable to do any of the things you used to find absorbing, it would be very strange if you did not react by getting agitated and trying to tell those around you how you felt.

Generally speaking, dementia is challenging because it is difficult for those of us without the condition to understand the world of PwD. Care homes for PwD should expect 'challenging behaviour' and accept it. Their staff should be trained and understanding. Their spaces should be aimed at people who are confused and whose behaviour is not 'normal'. These homes should not expect the people they care for to conform to the same daily pattern as the rest of the world – to wake in the morning, eat three meals a day, sit quietly in the lounge, accept personal care when specified and go quietly to sleep at night just because it is dark and this is what the rest of the world is doing. Specialised dementia care homes should specialise in caring for PwD – not in forcing those people to conform to a pattern which fits the convenience of the carers and the expectations of their families.

Dying from boredom

Although it is true that most PwD can find it hard to follow their previous interests and occupations, that doesn't mean that they are truly happy to sit quietly and do nothing. Many PwD become very bored and much difficult behaviour stems from abject boredom. Most care homes have an activities manager whose job it is to arrange entertainment and activity sessions and this can be a very challenging job. Often the activities manager is expected to take a group of people of vastly differing abilities and arrange something during the 'activity time' to keep them quiet and fulfilled whilst other staff are able to take a break.

It is quite impossible for one person to manage an activity session for a disparate group of people which will keep them all equally well entertained, so they often are forced to fall back on something like a TV film afternoon, coffee morning, group singing, or reminiscence session which the majority of the group will be able to enjoy at least in part. The rest will fall asleep, become disruptive and have to be removed to their room, or refuse to become involved.

This is not meant to disparage the efforts of activity managers in general. Most of them care about their job, want to do their best by those they have charge of, and spend time and trouble thinking of good ways to fill the 'activity hours'. However, those of us living independently don't usually have a set 'activity time'. We do the things we enjoy doing at the times we want to do them. We also do not need the help of others in order to entertain ourselves, although we may well interact with others in the course of our hobbies and pastimes. So, we are back again to the staffing problem – at many times of the day PwD need one-to-one help and support and with that support they can continue to carry out many activities – without it they cannot. Most of those living in care homes are condemned to a slow death from sheer boredom.

REFERENCES

1. Estes CL, Swan JH, Gerard LE. Dominant and competing paradigms in gerontology: Towards a political economy of ageing. *Ageing and Society* 1982; 2(02): 151-64.

2. Walker A. Towards a political economy of old age. *Ageing and Society* 1981; 1(01): 73-94.

3. *The Economist*. The demographic time-bomb. *The Economist*, Aug 27, 2008.

4. Department of Health. Living Well With Dementia: A National Dementia Strategy. GOV.UK; 2009. https://www.gov.uk/government/publications/living-well-with-dementia-a-national-dementia-strategy (accessed 23 July 2017).

5. Ahmad S, Orrell M, Iliffe S, et al. GPs' attitudes, awareness, and practice regarding early diagnosis of dementia. *British Journal of General Practice* 2010; 60(578).

6. Greaves I, Jolley D. National Dementia Strategy: well intentioned– but how well founded and how well directed? *British Journal of General Practice* 2010; 60(572): 193-98.

7. Koch T, Iliffe S. Rapid appraisal of barriers to the diagnosis and management of patients with dementia in primary care: a systematic review. *BMC Family Practice* 2010; 11(1): 52.

8. Milne A. Dementia screening and early diagnosis: The case for and against. *Health, risk & Society* 2010; 12(1): 65-76.

9. Burns A, Buckman L. *Timely diagnosis of dementia: Integrating Perspectives, Achieving Consensus*. Timely Diagnosis of Dementia Consensus Group; 2013.

10. Ferri CP, Prince M, Brayne C, et al. Global prevalence of dementia: a Delphi consensus study. *The Lancet* 2006; 366(9503): 2112-17.

11. Erkinjuntti T, Østbye T, Steenhuis R, et al. The effect of different diagnostic criteria on the prevalence of dementia. *New England Journal of Medicine* 1997; 337(23): 1667-74.

12. Anthony JC, LeResche L, Niaz U, et al. Limits of the 'mini-mental state'as a screening test for dementia and delirium among hospital patients. *Psychological Medicine* 1982; 12(02): 397-408.

13. BMA. Dementia diagnosis incentive caution. *BMA* 2014. https://www.bma.org.uk/news/2014/october/dementia-diagnosis-incentive-caution (accessed 30 June 2017).

13a. Anderson E, Petersen S, Wailoo M. Health concerns and needs of traveller families. *Health Visitor* 1997; 70: 148-150.

14. Collins N, Blanchard MR, Tookman A, et al. Detection of delirium in the acute hospital. *Age and Ageing* 2010; 39(1): 131-35.

15. Wanless D, Forder J, Fernández J-L, Poole T, Beesley L, Henwood M, et al. *Wanless Social Care Review: Securing Good Care for Older People: Taking a Long-term View.* London: Kings Fund; 2006.

16. Dilnot A, Warner N, Williams J. *Fairer Care Funding. The Report of the Commission on Funding of Care and Support* London: Department of Health; 2011.

17. Foucault M. The subject and power. *Critical Inquiry* 1982; 8(4): 777-95.

18. Cacioppo JT, Hawkley LC. Social isolation and health, with an emphasis on underlying mechanisms. *Perspectives in Biology and Medicine* 2003; 46(3): S39-S52.

19. Demaerschalk BM, Wingerchuk DM. Treatment of vascular dementia and vascular cognitive impairment. *The Neurologist* 2007; 13(1): 37-41.

20. Brayne C. The elephant in the room – healthy brains in later life, epidemiology and public health. *Nature Reviews Neuroscience* 2007; 8(3): 233-39.

21. Campbell D. Care home residents deprived of liberty in record numbers. *The Guardian* 28 September 2016.

22. Chaufan C, Hollister B, Nazareno J, et al. Medical ideology as a double-edged sword: The politics of cure and care in the making of Alzheimer's disease. *Social Science & Medicine* 2012; 74(5): 788-95.

23. Hughes B, Paterson K. The social model of disability and the disappearing body: Towards a sociology of impairment. *Disability & Society* 1997; 12(3): 325-40.

24. Marks D. Models of disability. *Disability and Rehabilitation* 1997; 19(3): 85-91.

25. Brown P, Zavestoski S. Social movements in health: an introduction.

Sociology of Health & Illness 2004; 26(6): 679-94.

26. Nots FM. *Welcome to Our World: A Collection of Life Writing by People Living with Dementia*: London: Alzheimer's Society; 2014.

27. Bartlett R. The emergent modes of dementia activism. *Ageing and Society* 2014; 34(4): 623-44.

Chapter 9

Death and dementia

Summary

- The three main causes of death for people with dementia are pneumonia, heart disease and pulmonary embolus (lung clot).

- The location where death in dementia occurs varies considerably across Europe.

- It is known that people with dementia who die in hospital generally receive less palliative care and attention to spiritual needs than people without dementia.

- Many people with dementia fear the prospect of a living or social death before the final, physical one.

- Some carers experience an anticipatory grief of their loved one with dementia. This can have positive and negative effects.

- Using a lifespan perspective can help in diagnostic counselling for people with dementia.

- Dementia diagnosis can be used to prompt advance care planning and exert some influence over the circumstances of one's death.

I. (NOEL)
What is the reality of death in dementia?

Dementia is defined as a progressive neurodegenerative condition that inevitably ends in death. However, predicting death in any individual with or without dementia is always difficult and estimates of survival post-diagnosis vary widely between three and nine years.[1] Whilst population-based studies provide some indication of what influences survival in groups of people with dementia (PwD), they do not tell us how PwD die. What do PwD die of? Where do they die? And most importantly, what is their experience of death? We shall look at these questions in turn.

Cause of death in dementia

What actually causes death in people with advanced dementia? Some studies have looked at this question using information from death certificates and autopsy records of PwD. One study by Keene et al, examined biological events prior to death in dementia. In their study, PwD survived 8.5 years post-diagnosis and the three main recorded causes of death were pneumonia, heart disease and pulmonary embolus (or clot on the lung).[2] Most had entered institutional care (76%) and nearly 60% died in an incapacitated state associated with their severe dementia, that involved urine incontinence (73%), reduced ability to eat (58%), immobility (38%) and faecal incontinence (21%).[2] In another study by Koopmans et al, most patients who survived to the final phase of dementia died from dehydration or wasting away (cachexia).[3] Do these statistics reassure or alarm? Looking at these, I have my own reactions. If these numbers reflected the reality of my own death in dementia, I would fear things like incontinence and the idea that I could be offensive or a burden to those caring for me. Similarly, I would be worried by immobility for the same reasons.

Cachexia or fading away, however, does not disturb me; neither does death from a heart attack or pneumonia. This is probably due to my experience in medicine and that I know that these can be relatively painless exits from the world. What I would like is to have some say about *where* I died. I do not want to die in hospital, but rather at home or in my nursing home, and I imagine that many people would also prefer this. I think it is more important to die in a comfortable environment, and unfortunately hospital wards are often busy, chaotic and confusing places for PwD to experience. I would not want fear and confusion to be my last sensations on earth.

Where do people with dementia die?

The place where PwD die does vary around the world. Most Americans who die of their dementia, die in their nursing homes.[4] In Europe, the picture is more mixed. The vast majority of people in the Netherlands whose death was dementia-related died at home with only a small group dying in hospital (92% versus 3%), whilst in Wales only 50% died in nursing homes and nearly the same (46%) died in hospital.[5] It is thought that good staffing in nursing homes, such as in the Netherlands, helps PwD avoid dying in hospitals.[5]

Quality of death in dementia

We have looked so far at what causes death in end-stage dementia and where PwD die. But what is the experience of death? Are most dementia-related deaths, 'good deaths' or traumatic deaths, irrespective of where they occur? Although this question has only received research interest relatively recently, the answers to these questions are unfortunately not very positive.

It is known that PwD who die in hospital receive less palliative care and less attention to spiritual needs than people who die without dementia.[6] Other research into the question of how PwD die has asked bereaved carers of their experience of their loved ones' death and what were positive and negative aspects in their witnessed accounts. And this has tended to focus on end-of-life care, given that dependency on care is a significant part of the last phase of dementia.

A qualitative study by Bayer examined family accounts of death in dementia, in a variety of settings. The quality of nursing care that relatives received dominated the collected narratives in the study. Distressing accounts of bad care, where PwD did not receive basic personal care and hygiene (such as assistance with eating and drinking) tended to occur in general hospitals.[7] Hospitals were also places where poor pain control and care planning with families were described. In their study, for people with end-stage dementia with more complex needs, NHS continuing care, which is free care for outside of hospital that is arranged and funded by the NHS, provided superior care to both nursing homes and hospitals. Of note, the demand for NHS continuing care is increasing and the sustainability is threatened by the increasing financial pressure on the NHS. The net public expenditure on continuing health care for older people, continues to increase year on year and is projected to rise from £2.25 billion in 2016 to £2.89 billion in 2022.[8]

Fear of living and social death in dementia

When examining the fear that people have of dementia, unpacking the concept of death is required. This is because I think PwD or their carers fear the possibility of a living death, or a social death, before the final, physical one. These feared states can be addressed to some degree using concepts of personhood and quality of life in dementia – namely, that personhood and quality of life are generally retained in dementia, irrespective of the stage of the illness, even if these may have different meanings from in our pre-morbid life. However, when life is viewed in narrow terms, and falls below a pre-morbid threshold of function and cognition, it may be viewed as a 'death'.

Part of the problem can be the lack of usual responses in people with severe dementia, so that carers may believe that 'only their heartbeat is left'.[7] I think that the fear of a living death in dementia will only be challenged when dementia is discussed more openly using other paradigms than the medical model, and we embrace more inclusive definitions of valued living. People with dementia only experience a social death if we allow it. And Kitwood would argue that the social death, or malignant alienation of PwD, is created not by dementia, but by the reaction of others to people with the condition.[9]

Anticipatory grief

One reaction that Mary and I have certainly witnessed over the years to PwD is one of anticipatory grief. Anticipatory grief is defined as any grief reaction occurring prior to the actual death of the person, rather than after. It has been thought that anticipatory grief may be a protective mechanism in that it gives the future survivor the opportunity to 'rehearse' and experience emotions attached to grief in advance of the bereavement.[10] For some family carers of PwD, anticipatory grief can exist for some years, related to the observed decline of the loved one after diagnosis.[11] What is written about anticipatory grief is usually written from the perspective of the family 'griever', and whether the phenomenon is more a reflection of carer burden and depression, which can complicate rather than simplify grief post death.[11]

My main concern is about the effect of anticipatory grief on the PwD. Even if anticipatory grief provides some kind of psychological function for helping an individual cope with feelings associated with future grief, it can have a negative effect on the PwD. If it is perceived strongly, it can act to reinforce the effect of social alienation described by Kitwood and contribute to an individual's sense of malignant social isolation and social death prior to a physical one.

My experience of anticipatory grief suggests it often has more to do with the carer's reaction to diagnosis, rather than the reality of the situation of the PwD. The corollary of this is that if catastrophic predictions of caring in dementia for the carer are challenged, and the carer burden addressed, then anticipatory grief can be diminished. If this is successful, then both the PwD and the carer can move on from the diagnosis. This then becomes a vehicle to concentrate on living in the here and now, rather than behaving as if their loved one has already undergone a social death. I am not saying that anticipatory grief is abnormal. I think it is completely understandable that when given a diagnosis of dementia, the mind will go where it wants, thinking about the implications of the disease. Thinking that life is pointless for a loved one with dementia is a common experience.[12] However, it is when this becomes a preoccupation that interferes with the ability to interact with person in the here and now, that this becomes a problem often bigger than the dementia itself.

Death by dementia – a lifespan perspective

In my memory clinics, I have found that incorporating a lifespan perspective in diagnosis counselling can be helpful. I started to incorporate this routinely into my practice after completing my gerontology degree, which examined the changing nature of the human life span, which I summarise briefly in Chapter 1. I frequently frame the diagnosis of dementia with a number of other contexts and use this kind of phraseology: *100–200 years ago, it is highly likely that none of us would be alive having this conversation due to infectious disease and many people dying in their 30s and 40s. It is a new reality of life that if you have done well to avoid cancer, heart attacks or strokes, then memory problems and dementias can be the next wave of difficulty. This is the catch of us living longer lives.*

I will often make a comparison here between the average life expectancy and the age of the patient, again to contextualise the dementia diagnosis in demography, but taking care not to sound flippant. I also often state here that *there is no proven link between memory loss and quality of life*and that *you don't need to have a perfect memory to be you.* I haven't encountered any instances where providing this kind of context to discussing a diagnosis of dementia has been poorly received. This is not given instead of more practical advice regarding lasting power of attorneys, driving advice or advanced care planning, nor does it displace a conversation regarding cognitive enhancers or other medications. Rather, it is an explicit acknowledgement of age being the biggest factor for dementia, and that for most people receiving a diagnosis of dementia, this is the catch in living longer. And it is important to remember that many people diagnosed with dementia, will die of other causes than the dementia itself. In a previously mentioned study, survival for matched controls without dementia, was 11 years, only four years beyond people with Alzheimer's disease.[1]

How should death in dementia be?

I think a good death in dementia is largely what constitutes a good death generally. A complete discussion of this is beyond the scope of this book and my expertise, although Mary has considerable experience with this. I can, however, suggest how

I think death in dementia should be and what obstacles exist to achieve this in the majority of people. People fear suffering, pain and indignity during death. The extra fear in dementia, I think, is dying alone, allied with the fear of being unable to communicate with both our family and our carers. An additional fear, which overlaps with the ideas of a social and living death, is of our minds departing well before our body does. If this is the case, what happens to the dying body? And will it be treated with dignity?

I think that we all hope that we can all die pain free, without fear, and in a dignified manner and in the place of our choosing. This is an aspirational death that not all of us will achieve but there has been a lot of good work by UK researchers and palliative clinicians to improve the death experience for those suffering from terminal disease. Individuals can also improve their future death by some basic advanced care planning.

This may help instil a sense of some influence over the circumstances of death, which otherwise feels totally uncontrollable. And this may be particularly helpful for PwD. Mapping out what should be done (or more importantly what shouldn't) in the event of a medical emergency, for example, can help ensure that people need not die needlessly in hospital. I would much rather abstain from the possibility of cardiopulmonary resuscitation or some other invasive medical possibility to ensure I can die in my (nursing) home in the event of me developing pneumonia in my late-stage dementia. This may in fact be one of the advantages of a dementia diagnosis: the opportunity to confront death more consciously, and in doing so, have some influence over the event. This is in contrast to others who die more suddenly, or as a result of unforeseen event such as a stroke or heart attack.

What else can be done to aid the process of a good death in dementia? Again, I think a lot of what we have said previously, about living well with dementia, can help us all die well with dementia. In particular, not defining ourselves in terms of complete independence and autonomy with crystal clear cognition. This means being open to the varied expressions of humanity, and understanding that one of the truest expressions of our nature occurs in the 'transaction' of care, both in the delivery of care and in the receipt of it. No matter how much individualism may be valued by society, interdependency underpins our social selves and society. The ability to accept care during life will make care before death easier and less distressing. Accepting that life and death can be messy is also important. We enter the world in a plume of biological mess and may exit the same way. We can try to antisepticise our lives between these two bookends of life, but we will be inevitably reminded that the processes of living and dying are not tidy ones.

On a less existential level, the socio-economic circumstances of people's lives will reflect the circumstances of their death. Although dementia is a very democratic illness and affects people of all socioeconomic groups, and healthcare in the UK is (currently) free, social care costs money. There is no doubt that if people can afford care in a good home during life, this may translate to good end of life care, without recourse to care in hospital. And if a person has money, he or she will have more freedom in what type of care he or she can broker, including end of life care, but only if he or she has considered death and planned for this accordingly. Mary will now talk more about this. How can one think ahead and pragmatically plan for, and improve, one's death experience?

II. (MARY)

Dementia is a progressive condition and the end-stage is death. Many PwD die with dementia not from the dementia – that is they die from another condition, perhaps a chest infection or as the result of a fall resulting in a broken hip, and it is tempting to consider these incidents as merciful, since end-stage dementia is very upsetting to witness. Few people with late-stage dementia die at home. A diagnosis of dementia then is an opportunity to come face to face with our own mortality – and that of those we love. It may not be an opportunity everyone wants to embrace, but in some ways this diagnosis gives us all a chance to accept our mortality, and if desired, to plan for how we would like our own end of life to be. I have written extensively about end of life in other books,[14,15] including chapters on dying with dementia and, interestingly, readers have mentioned that although they found the subject difficult to face, most have been strengthened by the experience of considering their own end and have achieved some measure of peace from doing so.

It is still frequently the case that a diagnosis is received late – that is after the disease which causes dementia has already progressed and the symptoms are obvious and already disabling. This may mean that those who have been diagnosed with dementia are often unable to view their own future or to plan ahead, and thus the burden of facing the decisions about end of life falls upon the main carer and the family of the person with the diagnosis. A timely diagnosis can be more upsetting in that the person diagnosed will be in a position to understand, and be aware of the prognosis, but it does give the opportunity for them to take control and be active in planning their dementia 'journey' and its inevitable end.

Practical matters

There are practical matters to be considered of course, and it is unfortunate that sometimes these are seen to be the only considerations, or at least to be paramount in the minds of some medical professionals. I have personally refused to distribute 'Information packs' at diagnosis which have as their first page a 'Do Not Resuscitate Request', and my grounds for this are simple. These practical matters should certainly be discussed, but they should be approached sensitively and preferably not at the same time as a diagnosis is given. When I have supported people at the point of diagnosis I have found that practical matters are often at the forefront of planning but at this stage they revolve around such things as power of attorney, making a will and applying for financial benefits as appropriate. These are all important matters – some, such as making a will and giving power of attorney have to be tackled without delay, as no one can do either of these things unless they are deemed to have 'capacity' – that is, the mental capacity – to do them.

Giving power of attorney brings many emotions to the fore (sometimes more than the making of a will), in that this is the moment when we have to consider whom we most trust to attend to our affairs if we are no longer able to manage them ourselves. The 'most trusted person' is not always the most obvious. Interestingly, many people do not give power of attorney to their life partner but rather to a child or children. Many people who have just been diagnosed with dementia still have capacity to understand what giving power of attorney to another means, and they will be able to do this even if someone else has to undertake the complications of completing forms and filing the relevant papers. The ability to actually manage day-to-day financial matters is often one of the things which is lost early in dementia, so I always advise people to attend to drawing up a power of attorney as soon as possible after diagnosis if this has not already been done.

Thinking ahead

Often people will still shy away from considering other end of life decisions but I would suggest that the final days of your life surely deserve full consideration. None of us know for sure when our final life moments will happen, but the odds are that when they take place there will be no free time to consider important matters at that stage. End of life is about more than just decisions concerning when and in what circumstances to resuscitate. We can, each one of us, write down how we want our last days to be. We can all make time to discuss this with our families if they will allow that discussion. For example – would we prefer to die at home (wherever that home will be) or in hospital or perhaps in a hospice? Do we want active efforts to be made to keep our body alive at all costs, or are there circumstances in which we would prefer to be left to a peaceful end – the modern expression is 'allow natural death' (AND)? Do we consider it more important to be without pain at the end or to have a clear mind? (The two may sometimes be mutually exclusive). Would we like family to be with us or perhaps just a single loved one?

There are also considerations after end of life – organ donation perhaps or leaving one's body for research purposes, burial or cremation, funeral (religious or otherwise) or perhaps a 'life celebration'. Some people like to write down the songs and readings they would like at their funeral or life celebration and their wishes about how much money should be spent on this ceremony. It is possible to make our feelings clear about all these matters and there are valid ways to do this. Advance directives (or an advance decision, or living will) can be drawn up, which make clear what actions a person specifies should be taken for their health if they are no longer able to make decisions for themselves because of illness or incapacity. A health and welfare power of attorney can be given to allow someone else to make these decisions on our behalf.

Anyone can write an advance statement, which is simply an expression of what they would *like* to happen at end of life. A useful and simple document which incorporates wishes and preferences is the *This is me* card available from the Alzheimer's

Society. I have written about the practicalities of arranging these documents elsewhere but the important thing is to make your wishes clear – write them down and keep your document where others can easily find it.

Difficult conversations

A diagnosis of dementia is a time to rethink our priorities in these areas and to attempt to establish the feelings and wishes of the person who has been diagnosed. We should be careful at this stage not to attribute our own feelings about these matters to a parent, a life partner or a close relative. Just because the gradual loss of cognition fills you with dread, and you consider that you 'would rather be dead than demented', does not mean that this is how your loved one feels. Feelings can change over time and even if in the past the person you are caring for expressed certain wishes there is no certainty that they still feel the same. Indeed, a PwD may feel quite happy and contented with life and be unaware of the feelings of sadness and despair experienced by their carer. They may still feel that life is very worth living – even reduced as it is. But they may not and it may be that they are frustrated, angry and despairing, and genuinely believe that their life is not worth living. Conversely the carer – especially if a lifelong partner – may wish to prolong life at all costs.

If a PwD is admitted into a residential care home, then end-of-life wishes should be ascertained and included in the care plan. The care plan should also be regularly reviewed. If you are the main supporter for a PwD it is perfectly in order for you to inform the care staff about end-of-life wishes if no enquiry is made about this, and it is a good idea to make sure the care plan does include them. Similarly, on admission to hospital this information should be made clear. These conversations can be difficult and it is easy for the care home or hospital staff to omit them. If the person you care for has firm wishes, make sure that they are recorded, and, as much as possible, acted upon.

Establishing feelings and wishes

Establishing end-of-life wishes can be a very important part of caring, and if discussing these matters after diagnosis is difficult, carers can at least be sure that they are doing an important and loving thing. Sometimes it is very difficult for PwD to make their wishes known. An important factor concerning this ability in dementia is the loss of the ability to foresee or understand the consequences of one's actions or even to think clearly about the future. People with dementia have a tendency to exist 'in the now' and may find it very difficult to engage in discussion about a theoretical future. This means that their feelings about end of life may have to be inferred.

People with dementia may use expressions such as: 'It's awful' or 'There is nothing left' or 'I'm angry' when asked how they are and this can be indicative. Others will answer 'I'm fine' or 'I feel ok' or 'Very well' to the same question. People who rail over a particular episode or restriction (losing their driving licence say, or not being allowed to walk out alone) are more likely to be unhappy about their general situation and simply using that point to express this unhappiness and anger. They may also be deliberately uncooperative during routine memory tests. In contrast, some people seem to passively accept help from their carer, be amused at or simply unaware of difficulties when answering memory questions, and give upbeat answers to questions about their daily living abilities. These differences in behaviour give us valuable clues as to how worthwhile people may find their present lives.

Living the life we want

This chapter is not just about end of life. A diagnosis of dementia also gives an opportunity to review our past life and to consider whether there are things we would still like to achieve and – most importantly – how we would like the remainder of our life to be. Carers who learn about the realities of dementia, about how it affects the mind and in particular the emotions – these carers are in a position to establish a good environment for the person they care for, and to ease the way through the loss of ability and the frustrations and pain of cognitive deterioration. People with dementia who accept their diagnosis and willingly accept support and help have an easier time.

The truth is that these types of carers and these types of PwD are few. Most carers get tired, dispirited, lonely and upset and many PwD are angry, frustrated, miserable and determined to reject help. These are facts and they may be hard to face up to. Media advertisements and upbeat articles that constantly show smiling happy PwD and carefree carers indulging in jolly sing-alongs or pleasant reminiscence do nothing to help those faced with the reality of what the diagnosis means. Still, the diagnosis can be seen as an opportunity. If we now know that our life with the one we love is restricted in length, there is at least the possibility of making the time that is left a time of calm pleasure and enjoyment of shared experience.

It may not be easy – and given the symptoms and inherent problems of dementia it is unlikely that our plans will always develop as we wish, but having a plan and a determination to implement it at least gives a goal and can make us feel more in control. The onus here is more often on the carer because the person with dementia is now more and more under the sway of wayward emotions and progressively less able to control his or her destiny. There are still many experiences that can be shared and enjoyed but this enjoyment will always rely on acceptance and understanding of the dementia, and can be helped tremendously by a shared family responsibility and support and acceptance from the local community.

Within families a great deal rests on the unity of purpose and genuine desire to support those most affected by dementia. There is often a complicated relationship between family members, and I am constantly surprised at how few families seem able to 'pull together' with the aim of making life easier for the PwD and the main carer. Few people seem able to set their ego aside and consider solely the good of another – which is to say that there are surprisingly few saints amongst us. In the same way, local communities may find it difficult to bear the disruption to their own routine, the loss of a good companion, the inconvenience when a previously good neighbour becomes a needy or aggressive nuisance.

There is no easy answer which will help with acceptance. But any of us might find this easier if we could place ourselves in the shoes of the PwD and feel the powerlessness, the frustration and the final apathy that is the result of cognitive loss. All the present initiatives concerning dementia friends, dementia-friendly buildings and neighbourhoods, information and support courses for carers and peer support groups are helping. It is also true that there are many still struggling along with minimum support due to lack of knowledge of available resources. Every health and social care professional should be aware of this and be prepared to not only 'signpost' those needing support and help but actively guide them to achieve the level they feel they need.

When the end comes

Unfortunately, the final days of life often come in an unexpected manner. We would all like to imagine a final peaceful 'drawing to a close' of life perhaps surrounded by loved ones, well cared for and pain free. The actualities can be quite different. Perhaps a fall or an infection is followed by an emergency admission to hospital and a fast deterioration. Sometimes residential care homes are so worried about possible accusations of neglect or mismanagement that residents at the end of their life are admitted to hospital instead of being cared for in the surroundings they are used to.

As I have pointed out, there may not be time to consider wishes and advanced plans in these circumstances, although where these have been discussed and recorded it is more likely that they will be adhered to. Hospitals are generally bad places to die (they are designed to care for and cure), and privacy and peace and calm are rarely obtained there. The Alzheimer's Society publication *My Life Until The End – Dying Well With Dementia* notes that 'care of patients in hospital is still largely crisis driven which means that end of life care can often be poor'.[13] Nevertheless, my experience is that families who have discussed end of life, and who have planned and considered ahead, often feel more comfortable about events leading up to death even if things have not turned out the way they had planned.

REFERENCES

1. Fitzpatrick AL, Kuller LH, Lopez OL, et al. Survival following dementia onset: Alzheimer's disease and vascular dementia. *Journal of the Neurological Sciences* 2005;229:43-49.

2. Keene J, Hope T, Fairburn CG, et al. Death and dementia. *International Journal of Geriatric Psychiatry* 2001;16(10):969-74.

3. Koopmans RT, van der Sterren KJ, van der Steen JT. The 'natural'endpoint of dementia: death from cachexia or dehydration following palliative care? *International Journal of Geriatric Psychiatry* 2007;22(4):350-55.

4. Mitchell SL, Teno JM, Miller SC, et al. A national study of the location of death for older persons with dementia. *Journal of the American Geriatrics Society* 2005;53(2):299-305.

5. Houttekier D, Cohen J, Bilsen J, et al. Place of death of older persons with dementia. A study in five European countries. *Journal of the American Geriatrics Society* 2010; 58(4): 751-56.

6. Sampson EL, Gould V, Lee D, et al. Differences in care received by patients with and without dementia who died during acute hospital admission: a retrospective case note study. *Age and Ageing* 2006; 35(2): 187-89.

7. Bayer A. Death with dementia – the need for better care. *Age and Ageing* 2006; 35(2): 101-02.

8. Wittenberg R, Hu B, Comas-Herrera A, Fernandez J-L. *Care for Older People: Projected Expenditure to 2022 on Social Care and Continuing Health Care for England Older Population.* Nuffield Trust; 2012.

9. Kitwood T. Dementia reconsidered: the person comes first. In: Katz J, Peace S, Spurr S (eds) *Adult Lives: A Life Course Perspective.* Bristol: Policy Press; 2011: 89.

10. Sweeting HN, Gilhooly ML. Anticipatory grief: A review. *Social Science & Medicine* 1990; 30(10): 1073-80.

11. Garand L, Lingler JH, Deardorf KE, et al. Anticipatory grief in new family caregivers of persons with mild cognitive impairment and dementia. *Alzheimer Disease and Associated Disorders* 2012; 26(2): 159.

12. Sweeting HN. *Caring for a relative with dementia: anticipatory grief and social death.* University of Glasgow, 1991.

13. Kane M. *My Life Until the End: Dying Well with Dementia.* London: Alzheimers Society UK; 2012.

14. Jordan M, Kauffmann JC. *End of Life: The Essential Guide to Caring.* London: Hammersmith Press; 2010.

15. Jordan M, Kauffmann JC. *The Essential Guide to Life After Bereavement.* London: Jessica Kingsley Publishers; 2013.

Chapter 10

The future of dementia

Summary

- We hope that in the future, the combination of technology, social reform and education will enrich the lives of millions of people living with dementia.

- The world will become more dementia-friendly if we are more willing to enter the cognitive realities of people with dementia rather than forcing them to conform to our world.

- If we can foster more holistic views of ourselves during life then we can be sure that our 'selves' remain preserved in the face of dementia.

- We need to have a mature debate about what we value in society, and how we can best care for its most vulnerable members, including people living with dementia.

- We can reclaim the D-word, educate people (and ourselves) about the true nature of dementia, and try to reduce fear about the condition.

I. (NOEL)

Ted's story

Ted has just returned from the local shop to pick up dinner for tonight. He could have the food delivered by drone, but he has always liked the evening ritual of walking to the shop, so his day planner schedules this activity for him. His spatial and temporal orientation are very poor, but his smart watch vibrates and tells him it is time to walk to the shop to collect dinner. He is very familiar with his smart watch, which his memory counsellor recommended to him 30 years ago, when it was forecast that dementia in later life was likely and it would be important to feel comfortable with wearing and using the device. It feels like his old i-phone. The smart watch also activates a LED light trail that guides him to the hallway and to put on his smart jacket, which has smart thermal material that can heat up or cool down with the ambient weather.

Outside, his neighbourhood has been designed with dementia in mind and has LED light trails to guide him to the local shop; the route is all on one level and clearly lighted the entire way. This was the result of cognitive disability legislation enacted 30 years ago, which required all new communities to include environmental modifications to facilitate a dementia-friendly environment. His smart watch also monitors his progress to the shop, and is equipped with GPS and also an accelerometer in case he falls. He consented to auto-monitoring by his day planner some years ago and also, specifically, that he could be referred to an on-duty assistance team if data suggested he had fallen, or that he was unable to find his way to his destination or home (eventually).

Chapter 10

Ted has always identified himself as a 'walker' (having worked outside most of his adult life) and walking is accepted as essential activity that displays and preserves his sense of self. Although the environment around him mitigates risks of falls and getting lost, both Ted and his support network accept both that he be allowed to walk and that there are risks associated with this.

At the local shop, he is greeted by Kirsten. She has worked there for a good number of years and knows pretty much everyone. She enjoys the early evening visits from Ted and generally knows what he is after. Ted's speech is poor, but she can work out what he needs either through non-verbal gesturing to what pre-made meal he would like, or what is selected by his smart watch based on an algorithm of previous preferences. If Kirsten is not about, and there is some confusion about what Ted would like, his smart watch connects to the shop's register screen by Bluetooth and lets the attendant know what he is after. Ted enjoys the ritual of the shop and walking about seeing the various displays of real and virtual food (that can be prepared), as well as interacting with who is about. Sometimes he may bump into a friend or two and enjoy a smile or non-verbal interaction, or he can choose to have an emoticon conversation on the visual interactive displays that line the shop and all public places.

Once home, and after dinner, Ted's daughter Sarah calls from Los Angeles. She has worked there for many years as her employer offered the best opportunities. She was initially very reluctant to accept a position so far from her dad, but was reassured by the policies and assistive technology in place that meant she could play a regular part in her father's life, even at such a distance. She calls generally each evening and her face will appear on the audio-visual wall of Ted's studio. Sometimes, she will use 3D Skype to make an 'appearance' and virtually visit her dad. If on some nights, she is unable to make a call, and if her father's smart watch monitoring of his vitals is interpreted by NEWS (Nido Electronic Wellbeing System) to indicate distress or increased worry, an interactive 3D hologram of Sarah will be projected and ask him what is wrong.

If he remains distressed, this will trigger the on-call local volunteer to arrive. Betty lives just two streets away, and is 82. She decided to enroll in the local volunteer scheme as any care that she volunteers results in an accrual of carer credits that will reduce the cost of her own care at a later stage, if she ever needs it. Apart from the sense of community this gives her, she finds it comforting that the same arrangements will be in place in the future if she should ever need them.

When Ted's dementia was diagnosed at 96, it was not a shock or concern to either of Ted or his daughter. Many of Ted's friends were not fortunate to have lived to his age; most died of cancer in their 80s. Ted and Sarah both received dementia and memory education at school and through their wellbeing sessions at the local wellbeing centre. As well as preventative information around diet, exercise and the importance of socialising, they also received information about memory and personhood. They both know that even if dementia progresses to an advanced stage, Ted will still be Ted, and that for most people in 2073, dementia is not an obstacle to enjoying a good quality of life.

Ted and Sarah know this at first hand as a friend, Sam, died of dementia last year. Despite losing the ability to speak, they enjoyed Sam's company in the later stages of his life. Sam would often believe he was back in London in 2017. Ted and Sarah used to enjoy his reality and spending time with him there. Sam's wife used to tell them of her experiences of her own mother's dementia around that time. And how, before care agencies were bailed out like the banks and renationalised, care had to purchased through a care broker.

Ted and Sarah were surprised that many people back then had to sell everything to afford basic care. They were relieved that their country had adopted a compulsory social insurance model, following Germany's lead, and people's care in later life was now heavily subsidised by the state. Ted and Sarah have used Ted's dementia as an opportunity to reflect on life and death, knowing that despite the advances in medicine that have abolished AIDs, and many other illnesses, we are all mortal. In adulthood, they had both taken wellbeing classes on 'our multiple selves' and knew that even if cognition and function fall, key parts of the self are robust in dementia. They both find this a helpful concept, as well as being offered other advice for facing dementia's challenges.

Improving the future of dementia

In Ted's narrative above, I have described a dementia utopia in the future where a combination of technology, social reform and education has improved the life of people affected by dementia. I hope that in 2073, the lives of people with dementia (PwD) might be like Ted's. In the absence of a 'cure', there are many ways that the experience of dementia can be improved. Although technology will take a more active role in the care, safety and maintenance of personhood in the future, changing our thinking and approach to dementia can make a real difference now.

We need to accept the rising prevalence of dementia as the sign of something good – namely, most of us living longer lives. Rather than living in fear of dementia, or in the hope that it never touches us, we should instead ask ourselves, how do we want our dementia to be? This then naturally leads to an earlier awareness and discussion of the issues affecting PwD.

In the future I hope there will be more willingness to use the biomedical model alongside other understandings of dementia. Illness narratives, in particular, remind us that dementia is a social experience, as well as a disease, that has many elements. Hopefully, society will become more open to different cognitive realities, and we will be more willing to enter the world of PwD, rather than making them conform to ours. Adopting a more playful response to reality, as we already do with children, would be a good starting point. I hope that we focus much more on maintaining personhood in dementia and become better at using the diagnosis, alongside rather than in front of the person. I also look forward to the time when mitigation of risk does not trump personhood. I hope that Kitwood's ideas and medical sociology can be introduced to medical and nursing students. And as a society, I hope we become less wedded to our strict hyper-cognitive definitions of ourselves, and the supreme importance of individualism. Instead, I hope we can adopt more flexible views of ourselves that are connected to others in a social web, and that even if memory fades, integral aspects of the self remain, preserved in the face of dementia.

I also wonder whether PwD would be better served using the concept of cognitive disability, as it is often the social and physical environment that disables PwD rather than the deficit in the individual. I really hope that the Dutch model of dementia-friendly communities that use clever physical environments, as well as decent staffing levels, take hold globally. I also hope that social input for PwD is accepted to be as important as any medication, and that the nonsensical division of health and social care interventions is removed. I hope that care, in general, assumes a greater status globally. We also need to have a mature debate about what we value in society and how we treat its vulnerable members. Although the prospect of a single 'bullet' or cure for dementia is intoxicating, we cannot let this divert attention away from reform of care systems and funding to better meet the needs of PwD. Other countries such as Japan, Denmark and Germany have made the state provision of accessible and affordable care to its older citizens a priority. But countries such as the UK seem more content to view care in dementia as a family and personal responsibility, where formal care must be brokered like a mortgage. This creeping commodification of care needs to be acknowledged and debated more widely.

Lastly, I hope that we decide what to do with the word 'dementia'. It has been a source of fear and dread for too long. We can either abandon it for something more clinical and less fearful, such as 'cognitive impairment'. Alternatively, we can reclaim the word, educate about the true nature of dementia (and ourselves), and try to reduce fear about the condition. Given that dementia is often associated with a fear of losing one's mind, the discipline of psychiatry may be best equipped to reduce the stigma of the condition, alongside a campaign to reduce the stigma of mental illness more generally. The use of Kitwood's phraseology 'rementia' alongside dementia may also help teach us that much can be done to reverse the social alienation that accompanies the condition. I remain optimistic that society will view dementia in a more enlightened way in the future and we will manage to deconstruct the fear surrounding the 'D' word. When this occurs, then, in the words of Susan Sontag, dementia 'will be partly de-mythicised ... without implying a fatalistic diagnosis or a rousing call to fight by any means whatever a lethal, insidious enemy'.[1]

II. (MARY)

The world of dementia is beginning to look a lot like the world of cancer. We understand now that dementia is just a global term for the symptoms displayed. There are many diseases (there are thought to be more than 200) which give rise to the symptoms of dementia. We are beginning to find successful ways to treat some of these diseases. For example, we now know that Korsakoff's syndrome can be treated with injections of B vitamins and by abstention from alcohol. The dementia resulting from the disease is thereby stopped from progressing, but the dementia symptoms are not 'cured'. It may be that in the future we will find ways to arrest the progress of dementia through the judicious use of drugs, but the hopes of a cure are indeed still out of sight and I feel, like Noel, that the constant media attention given to supposed wonder-drugs which turn out to be failures are shifting our attention away from the things that we, as a society, could be doing *now* to give help and hope to those whose lives are affected by dementia.

Community efforts

I have been at the forefront of support for PwD and their carers. Many are interested in the possibilities of a cure or of a medical advance which will alleviate their suffering, but many more are interested in what can be done to help and support them now to live their everyday lives with less stress, with more enjoyment and with more prospect of happiness. The finest moments in my support role have been when my clients have said that a suggestion, a piece of advice or a signposting to a service, have made a difference to the way they are able to live well *now* with dementia. The most satisfying times have been when I have been able to work together with a section of the community to provide or improve a service which will be of immediate benefit to people struggling to manage to live well with the disability of dementia. It has been most enlightening to see that those in the community who provide or enhance this service also gain great satisfaction from doing so, and also a new understanding of how seemingly quite small efforts make such a big difference.

The reality

Ted, Sheila and Phil's stories

Suppose 'Ted' wants to play golf as he always used to? It was a big part of his life. He would go down to the club for a game at least twice a week. When his dementia was in its early stages he could still play, as long as it was with an understanding friend at a quiet time of the day. His friend would keep score and redirect him when he became slightly muddled. But soon Ted's sense of direction became compromised. He didn't know in which direction to hit the ball. Other players became annoyed and impatient if he took too long to work out what he should be doing. The club was not unsympathetic. They suggested that Ted continue as a purely 'social' member. But somehow that wasn't enough. Ted no longer got the exercise he was used to and missed the company and companionship of former days.

Ted's neighbour Sheila used to enjoy going to the WI meetings every month. She volunteered to help in the gardens of a local attraction and met several friends at a nearby 'knit and natter' group in the local church hall. After she was diagnosed with dementia her driving licence was withdrawn. Some members of the WI volunteered to give her a lift to meetings, but often when they arrived Sheila had forgotten the date and was not ready. The volunteers got fed up with the confusion because it often meant they were late for meetings or missed them. The head gardener where Sheila volunteered couldn't cope when she made mistakes in her planting out or became distracted and wandered off in the middle of a task. Once she pulled up a whole bed of newly planted flowers thinking they were weeds! He asked her to stop coming. The knit and natter group was nearby so Sheila could walk there. She gradually lost the ability to follow a knitting pattern and had to ask for help from fellow group members more and more often. Sometimes she would mistakenly pick up someone else's knitting and spoil it by trying to work a few rows. After a while her fellow group members suggested she just come along for the 'natter' and skip the knitting. This worked for a while.

Phil, in the next street to Ted, lives with his wife Margaret and she helps him a lot. Because he lives with someone, Phil, even though he has dementia, is able to manage more easily than Ted or Sheila. Margaret is there from morning to night. She encourages him to get up in the morning, helps him with washing and dressing and makes sure he gets his meals on time. Often the two of them go out together shopping, meeting friends or visiting local places. However, Phil gets very confused if he is left on his own. Margaret cannot go out to see her own friends, conduct business at the bank or even keep a doctor's appointment without taking Phil along.

Ted would like to still have some kind of 'golfing experience' so that he feels an affinity with his past and he needs exercise and social stimulation. Sheila needs everyday help to get herself ready for appointments and to help her enjoy activities with others as she did before. She also wants to feel useful. Phil is helped a lot by Margaret and Margaret is happy to care for him. What she desperately needs is a little time to herself so that she can have a social life of her own. She would love to know that there was somewhere safe where she could leave Phil for a while if she has a doctor or dentist appointment.

Fulfilling the need

There are various services which purport to be available to those with cognitive problems and their carers. What most of these services lack is flexibility. It is impossible for the carer of a PwD to guarantee that they will be able to attend a service regularly without fail. Old age and frailty as well as declining cognitive ability may cause illness, accidents or falls which prevent attendance. The difficulties of rousing a PwD and having them ready to leave home early on any particular morning are many, so that fixed rules about transport and attendance may make the uptake of a service impossible for those who most need it. Some services also demand compliance in taking part with the activities offered, which many PwD will not do.

Of course, looking to the future and research aimed at the possibility of a 'world without dementia' are important. But as Noel put it, the 'brighter fantasy narrative' of a cure should not mean that we ignore the struggles of those living with dementia now. In concentrating on research rather than offering practical help and support, some charitable organisations are abrogating their responsibilities to people who are suffering *now* from the effects of dementia.

Dementia is not logical, it is not orderly and PwD are not all the same, nor do they all have the same needs. I feel that the best approaches are local community initiatives where care and support can be tailored as much as possible to those who need it. Examples of this would be: day care facilities which can offer a range of services from full day support to an hour of respite so carers can attend an appointment; clubs which have kindly members to help those who wish to keep up their membership as long as possible; local volunteer services who are not hidebound by rules about what they are prepared to do; local shopping areas where signage and shops are dementia-friendly; and neighbourhoods that are supportive of the needs of PwD without being intrusive.

People worry about the provision of the right level of support for those they are caring for, they worry about how to access this care and they worry about how to pay for it. There are not enough services which cater for dementia. When services are closed due to lack of uptake it is not because they are not needed. It is because they are inflexible, inaccessible or too expensive for those who need them. Where dedicated services are available, they may often be too costly for those who most need them. The average cost of day centre attendance at the time of writing is more than £50 per day and the cost of meals and transport to the day centre adds to this. The cost of employing a care-giver from a reputable agency to help someone with dementia with personal care is upwards of £17 per hour and if a PwD cannot wash or dress themselves, they need this help *every day* (weekends and Bank holidays included!).

State funding is not free – money for health and social care comes out of the purse of every tax payer so it is difficult to argue that provision of this kind should be free, but the iniquity of suggesting that dementia is a social problem rather than a health problem, when we know that the causes of dementia are physical disease, needs to be addressed. I am in agreement with Noel when he says that 'the biggest real source of stress to PwD and their families after diagnosis, is not the absence of a magic bullet or cure, but the worry about the provision of future care.'

The initiatives which are happening now in the UK, to make dementia-friendly communities, dementia-friendly high streets, dementia-friendly buildings and towns, are good beginnings. However, we should all be thinking about the question posed in the first chapter of this book: How do you want your dementia to be? We might like to consider that in working for 'dementia-friendly communities' now we are working for a better future for ourselves. The odds are high that anyone reading these words will develop dementia in due course. What can you do to improve the experience of *your* dementia?

REFERENCES

1. Sontag S. *Illness as metaphor and AIDS and its metaphors*: New York: Macmillan; 2001, page 87.

Useful Resources

POSTS AND ARTICLES

Alive inside
https://m.youtube.com/watch?v=NKDXuCE7LeQ

Caddell LS, Clare L. The impact of dementia on self and identity: A systematic review. *Clinical Psychology Review* 2010; 30(1): 113-126.

Kontos PC. Ethnographic reflections on selfhood, embodiment and Alzheimer's disease. *Ageing and Society* 2004; 24(6): 829-849.

Perry J. Expanding the dialogue on dementia: (Re)positioning diagnosis and narrative. *Can J Nurs Res* 2005; 37(2): 166-180.

Kitwood T. *Dementia Reconsidered: the Person Comes First.* Milton Keynes: Open University Press 1997: 89.

Livingston G, Sommerlad A, Orgeta V, Costafreda SG, Huntley J, Ames D, Ballard C, Banerjee S, Burns A, Cohen-Mansfield J, Cooper C. Dementia prevention, intervention, and care. *The Lancet.* 2017 Jul 19. http://press.thelancet.com/dementia.pdf

BOOKS

Jordan M. *The Essential Guide to Avoiding Dementia.* Hammersmith Books Limited (2013)

Jordan M. *The Essential Carer's Guide to Dementia*. Hammersmith Books Limited (2014)

Snowden D. *Aging with Grace* Fourth Estate (1998). (This is old and now out of print but it is still the longest study conducted of a single aging population and well worth reading.)

Gawande A. *Being Mortal*. Profile Books Ltd (2015). (Not strictly about dementia but says significant things about ageing, medical models and dying.)

Two books about the often neglected, spiritual side of dementia:

Treloar A. *Dementia – Hope on a Difficult Journey*. Redemptorist Publications (2016). (Although specifically written from a catholic viewpoint, this book discusses the spiritual side of dementia with great delicacy.)

Jewell A. *Spirituality and Personhood in Dementia*. Jessica Kingsley Publishers (2011).

Index

Abbreviations:
PwD, people with dementia.

Index

Index

Index

Other books by Mary Jordan

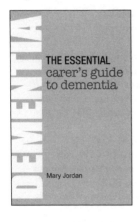

The Essential Carer's Guide to Dementia

'It is reassuring to have access to a book like this which brings together a wealth of expertise in dementia care, both personally and professionally, and illustrates the points most effectively with real-world examples. The tone is calm and practical, and helps to instil a belief in the reader that it is possible to manage such a challenging role in a positive and empathetic way. '

Frances Leckie, Editor *Independent Living*

The Essential Guide to Avoiding Dementia – Understanding the risks

'With knowledge comes the prospect of control, appropriate action and the potential for solution. I am in no doubt that this books has the potential to change how countless numbers of people might otherwise have ended their lives.'

Professor Graham Stokes
Director of Dementia Care, BUPA

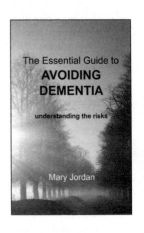

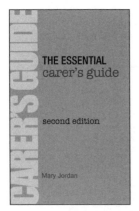

The Essential Carer's Guide – Second edition

'I found this book so helpful. So many things I worried about are addressed in this really practical book that just offers such brilliant advice. I picked up so many tips… plus it allayed some of my worries about simple things like personal hygiene and other areas. Really thorough and well written book and I dip in and out of it all the time.'

Amazon (Kindle) reviewer